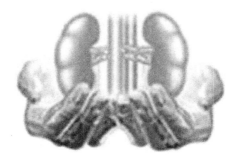

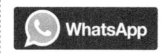

Complete Guide for Kidney Patients

Save Your Kidneys

Second Edition

Comprehensive Information About
Prevention and Treatment of Kidney Diseases

Edgar V. Lerma

MD, FACP, FASN, FNKF

Chicago USA

Sanjay Pandya

MD, DNB (Nephrology)

Rajkot, India

Elizabeth Angelica Lapid-Roasa

MD, FPCP, FPSN

Manila, Philippines

Coralie Therese C. Dioquino-Dimacali

MD, FPCP, FPSN

Manila, Philippines

Save Your Kidneys

Publisher

Samarpan Kidney Foundation,
Samarpan Hospital, Bhutkhana Chowk,
Rajkot 360002(Gujarat, India)
E-mail: saveyourkidney@yahoo.co.in

First edition: 2012
Second edition: 2015

Authors

Edgar V. Lerma, MD, FACP, FASN, FNKF
University of Illinois at Chicago College of Medicine, Chicago (Illinois, USA)

Sanjay Pandya MD, DNB (Nephrology)
Samarpan Hospital, Bhutkhana Chowk,
Rajkot 360002 (Gujarat, India)

This book is dedicated to all patients with
kidney disease and their families.

Table of Contents

Part1: Basic Information about Kidney

Part 2: Major Kidney Diseases and their Treatment
Kidney Failure

Other Major Kidney Diseases

Diet in Kidney Diseases

Preface to Second Edition

In writing the first edition of "Save Your Kidneys," Dr. Sanjay Pandya sought to write 'a book that would provide basic understanding and guidelines to prevent common kidney diseases.' Contrary to common nephrology texts, this book is primarily geared towards the layman.

This second edition is the collaborative result of the work of physicians with interest in further empowering our patients and their families with knowledge pertaining to various issues pertaining to kidney diseases. It is divided into two parts. The first part deals with 'Basic Information about the Kidneys,' which allows the reader to become familiar with the normal structure and function of the kidneys and also introduces the use of several technical terms. The second part deals with more specific kidney ailments, e.g., acute kidney injury, chronic kidney disease, diabetes, dialysis and kidney transplantation, etc.

The last chapter which is the work of Dr. Pandya himself talks about 'Diet in Chronic Kidney Disease.' It must be noted that the recommendations may not necessarily be generalizable to all populations because of various unique cultural and ethnic differences.

There is also a Glossary and Abbreviation List that the readers may find very useful as they read through the text.

Consistent throughout the book, is the use of vernacular that is familiar to lay people. We believe that this is important in bridging the communication gaps between patients and their care providers that can sometimes be brought about by medical jargon.

I am particularly thankful to Dr. Pandya and Dr. Vaccharajani for giving me the opportunity to contribute to this edition. I am also thankful to my colleagues Drs. Coralie Therese Dioquino-Dimacali, Elizabeth Angelica

Lapid-Roasa, and Filipina Cevallos Schnabel for their contributions in the arduous task of editing this book.

"Think like a wise man but communicate in the language of the people."

- William Butler Yeats

EDGAR V. LERMA MD, FACP, FASN, FAHA, FASH, FNLA, FNKF
Clinical Professor of Medicine
Section of Nephrology
University of Illinois at Chicago College of Medicine
Associates in Nephrology, SC
Chicago, IL

Preface to First Edition
Let Us Prevent Kidney Diseases...

The book "Save Your Kidney" is an effort to provide basic understanding and guidelines to prevent common kidney diseases.

In the last few decades there has been a dramatic and alarming increase in the incidence of kidney diseases. Chronic kidney disease is common and incurable. Awareness of the causes, symptoms and measures for prevention of these kidney ailments is the best way to counter this disturbing increase. This book is our humble attempt to provide that significant information to a layman in simple words.

Early diagnosis and treatment of this disease is beneficial as it provides long term benefits at low cost. Due to lack of awareness, very few people recognize signs and symptoms indicating a possibility of kidney disease, resulting in hazardous delay in early diagnosis. Treatment of advanced stage of chronic kidney disease such as dialysis and kidney transplantation is prohibitively expensive and in a country like India only less than 10% of patients can afford it. Hence early diagnosis and treatment remains the only and the most feasible option to decrease escalating cases of chronic kidney disease in our country.

When diagnosis reveals that a person is suffering from kidney disease, the patient and his family naturally become seriously worried. The kidney patients and their family members wish to know everything about the disease. But it is not possible for the treating doctor to provide a large volume of detailed information. We hope that this book will provide that missing link between the patient and the doctor. Anyway, it is rather helpful to have an informative book to read at a convenient time and refer to it as often as required. It provides all basic information about symptoms, diagnosis, prevention and treatment of different kidney diseases in simple and easy language. Details of selection and precautions in dietary recommendations for different kidney diseases are also included here. We need to emphatically and unequivocally state here that the information given in this book is not medical advice; it is for informational purposes only. Self medication or dietary modification by reading the book, without the advice of the doctor can be dangerous and is most certainly not recommended here.

This kidney guide will be useful not only to the kidney patients and their family but also to those at the risk of developing kidney disease. And, indeed, it will also be of educational importance for all those individuals who value awareness. Medical students, doctors, paramedicals are sure to find this book a handy reference guide.

We are thankful to Dr Gaurang and Dr. Susmita Dave, Mr. Ayaazkhan Babi and Neha Babi for their valuable suggestions and help to make this kidney guide easy to read and very clear to understand. We take great delight in making a special mention of our dear children Isha and Rohan who enthusiastically shared our sense of fulfillment and happiness in the preparation of "Save Your Kidney"

I hope the readers will find this book useful and informative. Sugestions to further improve this book are always welcome.

Wishing you all sound health,

Dr. Sanjay Pandya
Priti Pandya
Rajkot, India

About the Author of First Edition

SANJAY PANDYA, MD, DNB (Nephrology), Nephrologist

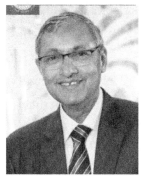 Dr. Sanjay Pandya is a senior nephrologist practicing in Rajkot (Gujarat - India). M.D. He earned his Doctor of Medicine (Internal Medicine) from M. P. Shah Medical College, Jamnagar (Gujarat) in 1986 and DNB Nephrology from the Institute of Kidney Disease and Research Center, Ahmedabad in 1989. From 1990 onwards he is practicing as Nephrologist at Rajkot (Gujarat), India.

Dr. Pandya is actively involved in kidney disease education. Kidney book for patients in English, Hindi, Gujarati and Kutchi languages is authored by him.

"Kidney Education Foundation" has been formed by Dr. Pandya with the mission to spread awareness amongst a large number of people for prevention and care of kidney disease.

With the help of a team of dedicated nephrologists from different parts of the world, educational books for kidney patients have been prepared in more than 20 languages.

In order to help maximum number of people and kidney patients in different parts of the world, www.KidneyEducation.com website has been launched by Dr. Pandya and his team. This website permits free download of 230 paged kidney books in more than 20 languages. This kidney website is very popular and has received more than 20 million hits in the first 60 months.

Free!!! 200+ Paged Kidney Book in 35+ Languages
Visit: www.KidneyEducation.com

About Authors/Editors of Second Edition

EDGAR V. LERMA, MD, FACP, FASN, FNKF

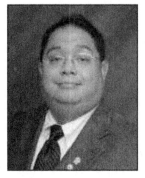 Dr. Edgar Lerma earned his Doctor of Medicine from the University of Santo Tomas Faculty of Medicine and Surgery in Manila/ Philippines. He completed his Residency Training in Internal Medicine at the Mercy Hospital and Medical Center and the University of Illinois at Chicago College of Medicine. In addition, Dr. Lerma completed a Fellowship in Nephrology and Hypertension at Northwestern Memorial Hospital, the Feinberg School of Medicine at Northwestern University, and the Veterans Administration (VA) Lakeside Medical Center in Chicago, Illinois.

Currently, Dr. Lerma is the Educational Coordinator for the Section of Nephrology at UIC/ Advocate Christ Medical Center in Oak Lawn, Illinois, USA. He holds the academic rank of Clinical Professor of Medicine with the University of Illinois at Chicago College of Medicine. He is also a member of Associates in Nephrology, S.C.

Dr. Lerma has many international publications at his credit. He has edited and authored many popular books such as Nephrology Secrets, Current Diagnosis & Treatment Nephrology & Hypertension, Renal Disease, An Issue of Clinics in Geriatric Medicine, Updates in Geriatric Nephrology, Current Essentials: Nephrology & Hypertension, Diabetes and Kidney Disease, Clinical Decisions in Nephrology, Hypertension and Kidney Transplantation, Kidney Diseases and Hypertension, Kidney Transplantation: Practical Guide to Management, Diseases of the Parathyroid Glands, Dyslipidemias in Kidney Disease, and Dermatological Manifestations of Kidney Disease.

ELIZABETH ANGELICA LAPID-ROASA, MD, FPCP, FPSN

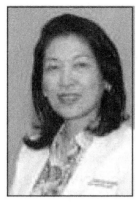

Dr. Lapid-Roasa obtained her medical degree at the University of Santo Tomas, Faculty of Medicine and Surgery in Manila, Philippines. She finished training as a resident in Internal Medicine and fellow in Nephrology at the University of Santo Tomas Hospital. She is a Diplomate and Fellow of the Philippine College of Physicians. She has served as a Board Examiner for the Philippine Specialty Board of Internal Medicine. She is likewise a Diplomate and Fellow of the Philippine Society of Nephrology and is a current member of its National Board of Trustees. She is also a Fellow of the Philippine Society of Hypertension.

Dr. Lapid-Roasa is an Associate Professor at the Faculty of Medicine and Surgery of the University of Santo Tomas. She teaches in the Departments of Physiology and Internal Medicine. She is the Chief of the Section of Nephrology of the UST Faculty and Hospital.

She has chaired the Clusters on Patient Care and Research of the PSN. She has contributed to the Asian Lupus Nephritis Network endeavors on the Asian guidelines and perspective on lupus nephritis management. She has been active in module development for basic immunology, renal physiology and clinical nephrology at the UST Faculty of Medicine.

CORALIE THERESE C. DIOQUINO-DIMACALI, MD, FPCP, FPSN

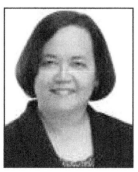

Dr. Coralie Therese Dioquino-Dimacali earned her Doctor of Medicine from the University of the Philippines College of Medicine (UPCM). She completed her Residency Training in Internal Medicine and Fellowship in Nephrology at the Philippine General Hospital where she served as Chief Resident and Chief Fellow, respectively. She also completed a Fellowship from the Foundation for the Advancement of International Medical Education and Research (FAIMER), Philadelphia from 2008-2010.

Dr. Dimacali served as President of the Philippine Society of Nephrology (PSN) from 2014 to 2015, after serving for several years as Officer and member of its Board of Trustees. She served as Chair of the Subspecialty Board of the PSN and was conferred a Life Fellowship to the PSN in 2008. She was also conferred a Special Award in Medical Education in 2006 by the PSN for her contribution in ensuring the quality of the Specialty board examinations and nephrology training programs in the Philippines. She is a most sought after lecturer with a special interest in nephrolithiasis, arterial blood gas, and fluids and electrolytes.

Currently, Dr. Dimacali is Associate Professor of Medicine and is Associate Dean for Academic Development of the University of the Philippines College of Medicine, a position she has held since 2012. She is also the recipient of the Dr. Victor Jr. and Maria Teresita Nañagas Professorial Chair.

FILIPINA CEVALLOS SCHNABEL, MD, MPH, FPSOHNS

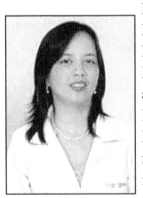

Dr. Filipina Schnabel is a graduate Doctor of Medicine of the University of Santo Tomas Faculty of Medicine and Surgery, Manila, Philippines. She has special interests in research and Public Health thus she pursued Masters of Public Health majoring in Epidemiology and Biostatistics at the University of the Philippines right after medical school. She took her residency in Otolaryngology-Head and Neck Surgery at the University of the Philippines-Philippine General Hospital and had her Fellowship in Laryngology, Voice and Swallowing Disorders at the Grabscheid Voice Center, Department of Otolaryngology, Mount Sinai School of Medicine in New York, New York. She further pursued Advance Laryngology at the Vanderbilt Voice Center in Nashville, TN. She held the position

Instructor V at the Faculty of Medicine and Surgery at the University of Santo Tomas teaching Preventive Medicine, Research, and Otolaryngology until her transfer to the United States. She was a consultant in Otolaryngology most especially Laryngology procedures at the Capitol Medical Center, The Medical City, St. Luke's Medical Center, East Avenue Medical Center and the University of Santo Tomas Hospital. She has published articles and lectured in Laryngology in several lay forums, study groups, conventions and conferences. She has been editing since high school and presently is one of the editorial staff of the Philippine Journal of Otolaryngology-Head and Neck Surgery. At present, she is a graduating Bachelor of Science in Nursing student of the East Tennessee State University and plans to pursue a Doctor in Nursing Practice.

How to use the book?

This book is into two parts

Part 1:

Basic details about kidney and prevention of kidney diseases are narrated. Each and every individual is advised to read this part of the book. The information provided can make a difference, as it prepares a lay man for early detection and prevention of kidney diseases.

Part 2:

One can read this part as per one's curiosity and necessity.

- Information about major kidney diseases, and its symptoms, diagnosis, prevention and treatment is discussed.

- Diseases damaging kidney (e.g. diabetes, high blood pressure, polycystic kidney disease etc.) and precautions to prevent it. Other useful information is also provided.

- Detailed discussion of diet for chronic kidney disease patients.

Information given in this book is not medical advice. Medication without the doctors advice can be dangerous.

Part 1

Basic Information about Kidney

- Structure and function of kidney.

- Symptoms and diagnosis of kidney diseases.

- Myths and facts about kidney diseases.

- Measures to prevent kidney diseases.

Chapter 1
Introduction

The kidneys are amazing organs that play a major role in keeping our body clean and healthy by flushing out unwanted wastes and toxic materials. Though their primary function is to remove toxins from the body, it is not their only function. The kidneys also play a crucial role in regulating blood pressure, the volume of fluid and electrolytes in the body. Although most of us are born with two kidneys, just one suffices to effectively carry out all important tasks.

In recent years, there has been a disturbing increase in the number of patients suffering from diabetes and hypertension that has led to a noticeable increase in the number of patients suffering from chronic kidney disease. This calls for better awareness and understanding of kidney diseases, their prevention and early treatment. Hopefully this book will address it aims to help the patient to understand kidney related diseases provides answers to frequently asked questions and be better prepared to deal with them.

The initial part of the book introduces readers to the kidney, its a vital roles in the human body, and suggests measures for prevention of kidney related diseases. The book deals with causes, symptoms and diagnosis of the dreaded disease, and also informs the readers about various treatment options that are available. In addition, a major portion of the book is devoted especially to matters concerning kidney patients and their families, as the authors deem this important part of patient care with kidney disease.

Know Your Kidney - Prevent Kidney Diseases.

A special chapter focuses on care to be taken during early stages of chronic kidney diseases and how to attempt to, slow down the progression of kidney disease to the point of requiring dialysis and even transplantation. Detailed useful information about dialysis, kidney transplantation and cadaver transplantation is also given separately.

To make the book a more complete guide for kidney patients, it include information about common kidney problems (other than kidney failure); myths and facts about kidney diseases; golden rules to avoid and prevent kidney diseases; tips about common drugs used by kidney patients and much, more.

Since diet is a very important area of concern and confusion for patients of chronic kidney disease (CKD), a separate chapter is devoted to this subject matter. It advises patients on precautions to be taken as well as selection of proper and adequate diet. The glossary at the end, explains all abbreviations and technical terms used throughout the book.

Disclaimer: Information provided in this kidney guide is for educational purpose only. Please do not indulge in any self diagnosis or treatment on the basis of the knowledge gained by the use of this book. You must always consult your doctor or other health professional for treatment.

The kidneys are among the most vital organs of the human body. Malfunction of the kidneys can lead to serious illness or even death. Each kidney has a very complex structure and function.

They have two important functions namely: to flush out harmful and toxic waste products and to maintain balance of water, fluids, minerals and chemicals i.e., electrolytes such as sodium, potassium, etc.

Structure of the Kidney

The kidney produce urine by removing toxic waste products and excess water from the body. Urine formed in each kidney passes through the ureter, flows into bladder before finally being excreted through the urethra.

- Most people (males and females) have two kidneys.

- The kidneys are located at upper and back side of the abdomen, on either side of the spine (see diagram). They are protected from damage by the lower ribs.

- The kidneys lie deep inside the abdomen so normally one cannot feel them.

- The kidneys are a pair of bean shaped organs. In adults, a kidney is about 10 cm long, 6 cm wide and 4 cm thick. Each kidney weighs approximately 150-170 grams.

- Urine formed in the kidneys flow down to urinary bladder and then through the ureters. Each ureter is about 25 cm long and is a hollow tube- like structure made up of special muscles.

- The urinary bladder is a hollow organ made up of muscles, which lie in the lower and anterior part of the abdomen. It acts as a reservoir of urine.

> **Location, structure and functions of the kidneys are the same in males and females.**

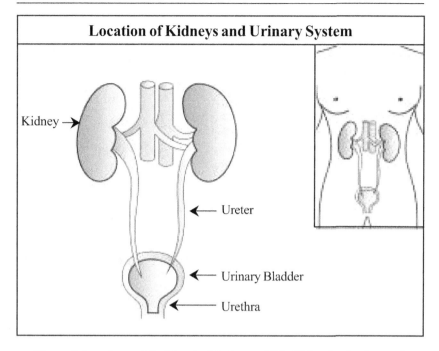

Location of Kidneys and Urinary System

Kidney →

Ureter

Urinary Bladder

Urethra

- The adult urinary bladder hold about 400-500 ml of urine; when filled to near capacity, a person feels the urge to pass urine.

- The urine in the bladder is excreted through the urethra during the process of urination. In females, the urethra is relatively short, while it is much longer in males.

Why are the kidneys essential for living?

- We consume different kinds and quantities and kind of food every day.

- The quantity of water, salts, and acids in our body also varies every day.

- The continuous process of converting food into energy produces harmful toxic materials.

- These factors lead to changes in the amount of fluid, electrolytes and acids in the body. The accumulation of unwanted toxic materials can be life threatening.

- Each kidney carries out the essential job of flushing out harmful and toxic by-products. At the same time, they also regulate and maintain the right balance and levels of water, acids and electrolytes.

What are the functions of the kidney?

Functions of the Kidney

- Removal of waste products
- Removal of excess fluid
- Balance minerals and chemicals
- Control of blood pressure
- RBC production
- To maintain healthy bones

The primary function of the kidney is to make urine and purify the blood. Each kidney removes waste materials, and other chemicals which are not required by the body. Important functions of the kidney are described below.

1. Removal of waste products

Purification of blood by removal of waste products is the most important function of the kidney.

The food that we consume contains protein. Protein is necessary for the growth and repair of the body. But as protein is utilized by the body it produces waste products. Accumulation and retention of these waste products is similar to retaining poison inside the body. Each kidney filters blood, and toxic waste products which are eventually excreted in the urine.

Creatinine and urea are two important waste products, that can easily be measured in the blood. Their "values" in blood tests reflects the function of the kidney. When both the kidneys fail, value of creatinine and urea will be high in blood test.

2. Removal of excess fluid

The second most important function of the kidney is the regulation of

Formation of Urine
Kidneys receive 1200 ml per min or 1700 litres/day of blood for filtration
↓
Glomerulus form 125 ml/min or 180 liter/ day Urine
↓
Tubules reabsorb 99% (178 liters) of fluid
↓
1-2 liter urine excretes waste products / toxins and extra minerals

fluid balance by excreting excess amount of water as urine while retaining the necessary amount of water in the body, that is essential for living.

When the kidneys, fail they lose the ability of removing this excess amount of water. Excess water in the body leads to swelling.

3. Balance minerals and chemicals

The kidneys play another important role of regulating minerals and chemicals like sodium, potassium, hydrogen, calcium, phosphorus, magnesium and bicarbonate and maintains normal composition of body fluid.

Changes in the sodium level can affect person's mental state, while changes in the potassium level can have serious adverse effects on the rhythm of the heart as well as functioning of the muscles. Maintenance of normal level of the calcium and phosphorus is essential for healthy bones and teeth.

4. Control of blood pressure

The kidneys produce different hormones (renin, angiotensin, aldosterone, prostaglandin etc) which help regulate water and salt in the body, which plays vital roles in the maintenance of good blood pressure control. Disturbances in hormone production and regulation of salt and water in a patient with kidney failure can lead to high blood pressure.

5. Red blood cells production

Erythropoietin is another hormone produced in the kidneys, it plays an important role in the production of red blood cells (RBC). During kidney failure, production of erythropoietin is decreased, which in turn leads to decreased production of RBC resulting in low hemoglobin (anemia).

This is the reason why in patients with kidney failure, the hemoglobin count does not improve despite supplementation with iron and vitamin preparations.

6. To maintain healthy bones

The kidneys convert vitamin D into its active form which is essential for the absorption of calcium from food, growth of the bones and teeth, and keep the bones strong and healthy. During kidney failure, decreased active vitamin D leads to decreased, growth of bones and they also become weak. Growth retardation may be sign of kidney failure in children.

How is blood purified and urine formed?

In the process of blood purification, the kidneys retain all necessary substances and selectively removes excess fluid, electrolytes and waste products.

Let us understand this complex and amazing process of urine formation.

- Did you know that every minute, 1200 ml of blood enters the kidneys for purification, which is 20% of the total blood pumped by the heart? So in one day, 1700 liters of blood is purified!

- This process of purification occurs in small filtering units known as nephrons.

- Each kidney contains about one million nephrons, and each nephron is made up of glomerulus and tubules.

- Glomeruli are filters with very tiny pores with the characteristic of selective filtration. Water and small-sized substances are easily filtered through them. But larger-sized red blood cells, white blood cells, platelets, protein etc. cannot pass through these pores. Therefore such cells are normally not seen in the urine of healthy people.

The kidney's chief function is to remove waste and harmful products and excess water in the form of urine.

- The first step of urine formation occurs in the glomeruli, where 125 ml per minute of urine is filtered. It is quite astonishing that in 24 hours, 180 liters of urine is formed. It contains not only waste products, electrolytes and toxic substances, but also glucose and other useful substances.

- Each kidney performs the process of reabsorption with great precision. Out of 180 liters of fluid that enters the tubules, 99% of fluid is selectively reabsorbed and only the remaining 1% of fluid is excreted in the form of urine.

- By this intelligent and precise process, all essential substances and 178 liters of fluid are reabsorbed in the tubules, whereas 1-2 liters of fluids, waste products, and other harmful substances are excreted.

- Urine formed by the kidneys flow to the ureters, and passes through the urinary bladder and is finally excreted out through the urethra.

Can there be variation in the volume of urine in a person with healthy kidney?

- Yes. The amount of water intake and atmospheric temperature are major factors which determine the volume of urine that a normal person makes.

- When water intake is low, urine tend to be concentrated and its volume is decreased(about 500 ml) but when a large volume of water is consumed, more urine is formed.

- During the summer months, because of perspiration caused by high ambient temperature, the volume of urine decreases. During winter months it is the other way round – low temperature, no perspiration, more urine.

- In a person with a normal intake of water, if the volume of urine is less than 500 ml or more than 3000 ml, it could indicate that the kidneys need closer attention and further investigation.

> **Too little or too much volume of urine formation, could be an indication that the kidney seeks attention and investigation.**

Chapter 3

Symptoms of Kidney Diseases

Symptoms of kidney diseases vary from person to person. A lot depends on the type of underlying disease and its severity. Symptoms are often, vague and non-specific, and therefore the disease is difficult to diagnose in the early stages.

Common symptoms of kidney diseases :

- **Swelling of the face**

Swelling of face, abdomen and feet, is a frequent presentation of kidney disease. One characteristic of swelling due to kidney disease is that it is usually noticed first below the eyelids (this is called periorbital edema) and is most noticeable in the morning.

Kidney failure is a common and important cause of swelling. But one needs to bear in mind that swelling does not necessarily indicate kidney failure. In certain kidney diseases, despite normal kidney function , swelling still occurs (e.g. nephrotic syndrome). Equally important, is the fact that swelling may not be seen in some patients despite significant kidney failure.

- **Loss of appetite, nausea, vomiting**

Loss of appetite, abnormal taste in the mouth and poor food intake are common problems faced by a person with kidney failure. With worsening of kidney function, there is increased level of toxic substances, which leads to nausea, vomiting and occassionlly, intractable hiccups.

- **High blood pressure - Hypertension**

In patients with kidney failure, hypertension is common. If hypertension occurs at a young age (less than 30 years) or blood pressure is very high at the time of diagnosis, the reason may be that of a kidney disease.

Swelling of face below the eyelids (called periorbital edema) is the most common symptom of kidney diseases.

- **Anemia and weakness**

Generalized weakness, early fatigue, poor concentration and pallor are common complaints of a person with anemia (low hemoglobin level). At times these may be the only complaints of a person in the early stages of chronic kidney failure. If anemia does not respond to standard treatment, it is essential to rule out kidney failure.

- **Nonspecific complaints**

Low back pain, generalized body aches, itching and leg cramps are frequent complaints in kidney disease. Retardation of growth, short stature and bending of leg bones are common in children with kidney failure.

- **Urinary complaints**

Common urinary complaints are :

1. Reduction in urine volume, is very common in various kidney diseases.
2. Burning sensation in urine (dysuria), frequent urination (frequency) and passing of blood or pus in urine are symptoms of urinary tract infection.
3. Obstruction to the normal flow of urine can lead to difficulty in 'voiding' (passing urine), and poor stream of urine. In severe conditions, complete inability to pass urine can occur.

Although a person may have some of the above mentioned symptoms and signs, it does not necessarily mean that the person is suffering from kidney disease. However, in the presence of such symptoms, it is highly recommended to consult the doctor and to rule out any possibility of kidney disease and other systemic illnesses by blood and urine tests.

It is important to remember that serious kidney problems may exist silently for a long period without significant symptoms and signs.

Rule out underlying kidney diseases if severe hypertension is detected at a young age.

Chapter 4
Diagnosis of Kidney Diseases

The old saying "A stitch in time saves nine" holds true for the treatment of kidney diseases. Chronic kidney disease (CKD) is not curable and if not treated can lead to end stage kidney disease (ESKD). As discussed in the previous chapter, a person with CKD can be asymptomatic, i.e. no symptoms of the disease may be apparent. However if diagnosis of kidney disease is made early, appropriate medical treatment can be rendered and progression to ESKD can be delayed or slowed. So whenever a kidney problem is even suspected, it is advisable to go for immediate check up and early diagnosis.

Who should get their kidneys checked? Who is at high risk for developing kidney problems?

Anyone can develop a kidney problem, but the risk is higher in the presence of :

- Symptoms of kidney disease
- Diabetes
- Difficult to control hypertension
- Family history of kidney disease, diabetes and hypertension
- Chronic tobacco consumption, obesity and/or elderly (above 60 years)
- Chronic intake of pain relievers, e.g., nonsteroidal anti-inflammatory drugs such as ibuprofen, naproxen
- Congenital defect of urinary tract

Screening in such high risk individuals helps in early detection and diagnosis of kidney disease.

> **Early stages of chronic kidney disease are usually asymptomatic, laboratory tests are the only way of detection.**

How to diagnose kidney problems? What tests are normally performed?

To diagnose different kidney problems the doctor takes a detailed history, thoroughly examines the person, check the blood pressure and then advises appropriate tests. Routinely performed and most useful tests include urine tests, blood tests and radiological tests.

1. Urine Tests

Different urine tests provide useful clues for the diagnosis of various types of kidney disease.

Routine urinalysis

- It is a simple, inexpensive and very useful diagnostic test.

- Abnormality seen in a routine urinalysis provides important diagnostic clues but a normal urinalysis does not necessarily rule out underlying kidney diseases.

- Presence of protein in urine (proteinuria) is seen in various kidney diseases. It should never be neglected. Presence of protein in urine can be the first, the earliest and the only warning sign of chronic kidney disease (and even of heart disease). For example proteinuria is the first sign of kidney involvement in diabetes.

- Presence of pus cells in urine may indicate the presence of urinary tract infection (UTI).

- Presence of protein and red blood cells (RBCs) provides diagnostic clues for inflammatory kidney disease (i.e. glomerulonephritis).

Microalbuminuria

Microalbuminuria means that a very small amount of protein is present in urine. This test provides the first and the earliest clue for the diagnosis of kidney involvement in diabetes. At this stage, the disease may be potentially reversible with proper and meticulous treatment.

Routine urinalysis is very important for the early detection and diagnosis of kidney disease.

Other urine tests

- **24 hour urine for protein:** In patients with the presence of protein in urine, this test is necessary to determine the total actual amount of protein lost in 24 hours. This test is useful to assess the severity of the disease and also the effect of treatment on the loss of protein.

- **Culture and sensitivity test:** This test provides valuable information about the type of bacteria causing UTI, and the choice of antibiotic selection for its treatment.It may take 48-72 hours to get the final results of this test.

- **Urine test for acid fast bacilli:** This test is useful to diagnose tuberculosis of urinary tract.

2. Blood Tests

Various blood tests are necessary to establish appropriate diagnosis of different kidney diseases.

• Creatinine and Urea

Blood levels of creatinine and urea reflects the function of the kidneys. Creatinine and urea are two by- products which are normally removed from the blood by the kidney. When the kidney function slows down, the blood levels of creatinine and urea increase. Normal value of serum creatinine is 0.9 to 1.4 mg/dl and normal value of blood urea nitrogen (BUN) is 20 to 40 mg/dl. Higher values suggest damage to the kidneys. Creatinine level is a more reliable guide of kidney function as compared to BUN.

• Hemoglobin

Healthy kidneys help in the production of red blood cells which contain hemoglobin. When hemoglobin is low, it is called anemia. Anemia is a common and important sign of chronic kidney diseases. However anemia can occur quite frequently in other illnesses. So anemia is not a specific test for kidney diseases.

Serum creatinine is a standard blood test used routinely to screen for and monitor kidney disease.

- **Other blood tests**

Different blood tests frequently performed in kidney patients include: blood sugar, serum albumin, cholesterol, electrolytes (sodium, potassium and chloride), calcium, phosphorous, bicarbonate, ASO titer, complement levels etc.

3. Radiological Tests

- **Ultrasound of the kidneys**

A kidney ultrasound is a simple, useful, quick and safe (no radiation exposure) test which provides valuable information such as the size of kidney and the presence of cysts, stones and tumors. An ultrasound can also detect blockage to urine flow in the urinary tract. In advanced stage of CKD or ESKD both kidneys may be found to be small in size.

- **X-ray of abdomen**

This test is useul for the diagnosis of calcium containg stones in the urinary system urinary tract.

- **Intra venous urography (IVU)**

IVU (also known as intra venous pyelography-IVP) is a specialized X-ray test. In this test, a radio opaque iodine containing dye (fluid which can be seen on X-ray films) is injected into a vein in the arm. This dye then passes through the kidney and gets excreted in to the urine. The urinary tract (kidneys, ureters and bladder) are rendered radio-opaque, and this allows visualization of the entire urinary tract. A series of X-ray pictures are taken at specific time intervals which give a comprehensive view of the anatomy of the urinary system. IVU can reveal problems such as stone, obstruction, tumor and abnormalities in structure and function of the kidneys.

In cases of advanced CKD, IVU is usually not recommended because the injected dye can damage the already poorly functioning kidneys. In

> **The most important screening tests for kidney diseases are the urinalysis, serum creatinine and ultrasound of kidney.**

kidney failure, excretion of dye during test may be inadequate. This test is also not recommended during pregnancy. Because of availability of ultrasound and CT scan, this test is used much less frequently nowadays.

- **Voiding cystourethrogram (VCUG)**

Voiding cystourethrogram - VCUG (previously known as Micturating cystourethrogram - MCU) test is most commonly used in the evaluation of urinary tract infection in children. In this special X - ray test, under sterile conditions, the bladder is filled with contrast medium via the urinary catheter. After the bladder is filled, urinary catheter is removed and the patient is asked to urinate. X -rays taken at intervals during urination show the outline of the bladder and urethra. This test is helpful to diagnose backflow of urine into the ureters, and up to the kidneys (known as vesicoureteric reflux VUR) as well as identifying structural abnormalities of urinary bladder and urethra.

- **Other radiological tests**

In special circumstances for the diagnosis of certain kidney diseases, other tests such as CT scan of kidney and urinary tract, renal doppler, radionuclear study, renal angiography, antegrade and retrograde pyelography etc. can be useful.

4. Other Special Tests

Kidney biopsy, cystoscopy and urodynamics are special tests which are necessary for the exact diagnosis of certain kidney problems.

Kidney Biopsy

Kidney biopsy is an important test useful in the diagnosis of certain kidney diseases such as glomerulonephritis, certain tubulointerstitial diseases, etc.

A kidney ultrasound is a simple and safe test used to assess the size, shape, and location of the kidneys.

What is kidney biopsy?

During a kidney biopsy, a small piece of kidney tissue is removed through a needle and examined under a microscope. Kidney biopsy is performed to diagnose the exact nature of certain kidney diseases, e.g. glomerulonephritis and certain tubulointerstitial diseases, etc.

When is kidney biopsy advised?

In certain kidney diseases even a detailed history, physical examination and routine tests are unable to establish proper diagnosis. In such patients, a kidney biopsy may provide additional information, which can establish the correct diagnosis.

How does the kidney biopsy help?

The kidney biopsy establishes specific diagnosis of certain unexplained kidney diseases, e.g. glomerulonephritis and certain tubulointerstitial diseases, etc. With this information, the nephrologist is able to plan effective treatment strategy and guide patients and their family about the severity and course of the disease.

By which technique is a kidney biopsy performed?

The most common method is via a percutaneous needle biopsy (usually performed in the radiology suite), in which a hollow needle is passed through the skin into the kidney. Another rarely used method is open biopsy which requires surgery (performed in the operating room).

How is a kidney biopsy performed?

- The patient is admitted in hospital and his consent is obtained.
- Prior to biopsy it is ensured that blood pressure and blood tests on blood clotting are within normal. Medications used for the prevention of blood clotting (e.g. aspirin and clopidrogel) is recommended to be discontinued for at least 1- 2 weeks prior to biopsy.

The kidney biopsy is a test performed to establish the diagnosis of certain kidney diseases, glomerulonephritis certain tubulointerstitial diseases etc.

- Ultrasound or CT scan is done to know the position of kidneys and to determine exact biopsy site.

- The patient is asked to lie face down – on his/her stomach with the abdomen supported by a pillow or towel. The patient is fully awake during the procedure. In small children the kidney biopsy is done under general anesthesia, so the child is not awake.

- After proper cleaning of the skin, the biopsy site is numbed with local anesthesia to minimize discomfort and pain.

- With the use of a hollow biopsy needle, 2 or 3 small thread like pieces are obtained from the kidney. These specimens are then sent to the pathologist for histopathology examination.

- After the biopsy, pressure is applied to the biopsy site to prevent bleeding. The patient is put on complete bed rest for 6-12 hours and usually discharged the following day.

- The patient is advised to avoid heavy work or exercise for at least 2-4 weeks after the biopsy procedure.

Are there any risks to kidney biopsy?

Like any surgical procedure, complications can occur in a few patients after kidney biopsy. Mild pain or discomfort over the puncture site and passing of reddish urine once or twice is not uncommon, but it usually stops on its own. In rare cases where bleeding continues, blood transfusion may be required. In extreme and very rare circumstances where by intractable severe bleeding persists emergency removal of kidney by surgery may become necessary.

Sometimes kidney tissue obtained may not be adequate for diagnosis (about 1 in 20). Repeat biopsy may be needed in such cases.

The kidney biopsy is usually performed with the use of a thin hollow needle with the patient in the fully awake state.

Chapter 5

Major Kidney Diseases

Kidney diseases are divided into two major groups

- **Medical diseases:** Medical kidney diseases such as kidney failure, urinary tract infection and nephrotic syndrome are treated by nephrologists. Patients with advance kidney failure need treatment such as dialysis and kidney transplantation.

- **Surgical diseases:** Urologists treat surgical kidney diseases such as kidney stones, prostate problems and cancer of the urinary tract by surgery, endoscopy, and lithotripsy.

- **How do nephrologists and urologists differ?**

  Nephrologists are experts in the treatment of medical kidney diseases, slowing progression of kidney diseases dialysis and kidney transplantation; whereas, urologists are experts in the treatment of surgical diseases, such as surgical removal of stones, tumors, kidney and prostate cancer, etc.

Major Kidney Diseases	
Medical	**Surgical**
Acute kidney failure	Stone disease
Chronic kidney disease (CKD)	Bladder and Prostate problems
Urinary tract infection	Congenital urinary anomalies
Nephrotic syndrome	Cancer

Kidney Failure

Significant reduction in the ability of the kidneys to filter and excrete

> **Acute kidney failure is a rapid loss of kidney function. With short term treatment kidneys usually improve.**

waste products and to maintain the electrolyte balance is called kidney failure. An increase in the values of serum creatinine and blood urea nitrogen (BUN) usually implies kidney malfunction and disease.

Kidney failure is usually divided into two types: acute kidney failure and chronic kidney disease (chronic renal failure).

Acute Kidney Failure

A sudden reduction or loss of kidney function is called acute kidney (renal) failure or acute kidney injury (AKI).The volume of urine decreases in the majority of patients with AKI. Important causes of AKI include intractable diarrhea, intractable vomiting, falciparum malaria, intractable hypotension, sepsis, certain medications (NSAIDs) etc. With proper medical treatment kidney function may be restored in most cases.

Chronic Kidney Disease

Gradual, progressive and irreversible loss of kidney function over several months to years is called chronic kidney disease or – CKD (chronic renal failure). In CKD, kidney function decreases rather slowly but continuously. After a long period of time, it progresses to a stage whereby, the kidneys stop working almost completely. This advanced and life threatening stage of disease is called the end stage kidney (renal) disease (ESKD/ ESRD).

CKD is a silent disease and often goes unnoticed. In the early stages of CKD, signs or symptoms are few and non-specific. Common symptoms of CKD may include generalized weakness, loss of appetite, nausea and vomiting, generalized swelling, high blood pressure, etc. Two most important and common causes of CKD are diabetes and hypertension.

> **Gradual progressive and irreversible loss of kidney function over a long period is called chronic kidney disease (CKD).**

The presence of protein during urinalysis, high creatinine in the blood and small contracted kidneys on ultrasound are important diagnostic clues of underlying CKD. The value of serum creatinine reflects kidney disease and this value increases progressively over time.

In the early stages of CKD, the patient needs appropriate medications and dietary modifications. There is no specific treatment which can cure this disease. One has to realize that as one gets older, the kidney function also decreases. Concomitant illnesses such as diabetes and hypertension, if uncontrolled can contribute to faster and progressive decline of kidney function, along with age.

The aim of the treatment is to slow down the progression of the disease, prevent complications and thereby keep the patient well for a longer period, despite the severity or stage of the illness.

When the disease progresses to an advanced stage (End Stage Kidney Disease) more than 90% of kidney function is lost (serum creatinine is usually more than 8-10 mg/dl). The only treatment options available at this stage are dialysis (hemodialysis and peritoneal dialysis) and kidney transplantation.

Dialysis is a filtering process to remove waste products and excess fluid from the body that may accumulate in the body when the kidney stops functioning. Dialysis is not a cure for CKD. In the advanced stage of CKD (ESKD), the patient needs lifelong regular dialysis treatment (unless kidney is transplanted successfully). Two methods of dialysis are hemodialysis and peritoneal dialysis.

Hemodialysis (HD) is the most widely used form of dialysis. In HD, with the use of a special machine, waste products, excess fluid and salt are removed. Continuous ambulatory peritoneal dialysis (CAPD) is

> **Dialysis is an artificial method of removing waste products and excess fluid from the blood when the kidneys have failed.**

another form of dialysis modality which can be carried out at home or at work place without the help of the machine.

Kidney transplant is the most ideal treatment option and the only curative treatment modality of end stage kidney disease (advanced stage of CKD).

Urinary Tract Infection

Burning and frequent urination, pain in lower abdomen and fever are common presentations of urinary tract infection (UTI). Presence of pus cells in urine test may suggest UTI.

Most of the patients with UTI respond well to appropriate antibiotic therapy. UTI in children needs special consideration. Delay or inadequate treatment of UTI in children can cause irreversible damage to the growing kidney.

In patients with recurrent UTI, it is important to exclude urinary tract obstruction, stone disease, abnormality of urinary tract and genito-urinary tuberculosis by thorough investigation. The most important cause of recurrence of UTI in children is Vesicoureteric reflux (VUR). VUR is a congenital abnormality, in which urine flows backwards from the bladder into one or both of the ureters, and up to the kidneys, instead of the other way around, i.e. from the kidneys towards the bladder.

Nephrotic Syndrome

Nephrotic syndrome consists of a constellation of findings namely: edema (swelling of feet), massive proteinuria (more than 3.5 grams protein in the urine per day), hypoalbuminemia (low albumin in the blood) and high blood cholesterol levels. Such patients can present with normal or elevated blood pressure as well as varying degrees of kidney dysfunction as measured by creatinine levels in the blood.

Delay in treatment and inadequate work up of UTI in children can cause irreversible damage to the growing kidney which can have dire consequences.

This disease shows varying responses to treatment so that it is important to establish the underlying diagnosis early on. A few patients may remain symptom free after discontinuation of the treatment but in most cases the disease recurs, i.e., there may be periods of remission alternating with relapses depending on the stage of treatment.

It is important to realize that the long term outcome is excellent in treated children with nephrotic syndrome. They live healthy lives with normal kidney function.

Kidney Stones

Kidney stones are common and important kidney problems. The kidneys, ureters and bladder are common sites where stones may be found. Common symptoms of having kidney stones are severe, unbearable pain, nausea and vomiting, blood in urine, etc. However, some people who have had kidney stones, even for a long time, may not have any symptoms (silent stone), at all.

For the diagnosis of stones, abdominal X-rays and ultrasonography are the most commonly used investigations.

Most of the small sized stones pass out naturally with urine by consuming increased amounts of liquids. If a stone causes recurrent severe pain, recurrent infection, obstruction of urinary tract or damage to kidney, its removal may be necessary. The ideal method for removal of the stone depends on the size, location and the type of stone. Most common methods for the removal of stones are lithotripsy, endoscopy (PCNL, cystoscopy and ureteroscopy) and open surgery.

As the risk of recurrence of stone is as high as 50 - 80%, increasing fluid intake, dietary restriction and periodic check up are necessary for all.

Kidney stones can exist without symptoms for years.

Benign Prostatic Hyperplasia (BPH)

The prostate gland is present only in males. It is situated just underneath the bladder and surrounds the initial portion of urethra. The prostate gland begins to enlarge after the age of 50. An enlarged prostate gland compresses the urethra and causes problems in urination particularly in elderly males.

The main symptoms of benign prostatic hyperplasia (BPH) are frequent urination (especially at night) and dribbling at the end of the urination. Examination by inserting a finger in rectum (digital rectal examination, DRE) and ultrasound are two most important diagnostic methods for BPH.

A large number of patients with mild to moderate symptoms of BPH can be treated effectively for a long period with medicine. Many patients with severe symptoms and very large prostate may require endoscopic removal of the prostate gland (TURP).

**BPH is the most common cause of
urinary symptoms in elderly males.**

Chapter 6

Myths and Facts about Kidney Diseases

Myth: All kidney diseases are incurable.

Fact: No, all kidney diseases are not incurable. With early diagnosis and treatment many kidney diseases can be cured. In the majority of cases, early diagnosis and treatment can slow or halt progression.

Myth: Kidney failure can occur if one kidney fails.

Fact: No, kidney failure occurs only when both kidneys fail. In most cases, affected individuals may not manifest any problem if one kidney fails completely, and in such cases, the values of blood urea nitrogen and creatinine in the blood tests may remain within the normal range. However, when both kidneys fail, waste products accumulate in the body and the raised level of blood urea nitrogen and creatinine in the blood tests may be indicative of kidney failure.

Myth: In kidney disease, the presence of edema suggests kidney failure.

Fact: No. In certain kidney diseases, edema is present, but kidney function may remain normal (e.g. nephrotic syndrome). One has to understand that edema is simply a manifestation of altered fluid mechanics in the body, and one of the common causes of such a manifestation, is kidney disease.

Myth: Edema is present in all patients with kidney failure.

Fact: No. Edema is present in the majority of patients with kidney failure, but not in all. A few patients do not have edema even in advanced stages of kidney failure. So the absence of edema does not necessarily rule out kidney failure.

Myth: All patients with kidney disease should drink a large amount of water.

Fact: No. Reduced urine output leading is an important feature of many kidney diseases. So water restriction is necessary to maintain water balance in such patients. However, patients suffering from kidney stone disease and urinary tract infection with normal renal function are advised to drink a large amount of water.

Myth: I am all right, so I don't think I have a kidney problem.

Fact: Most of the patients are asymptomatic (showing no symptoms) in early stages of CKD. Abnormal values in laboratory tests are the may be the only clue (e.g., microalbuminuria) of its presence at this stage.

Myth: I feel fine, so I don't need to continue treatment for my kidney problem.

Fact: Many patients with CKD feel very well with proper therapy, and so they may discontinue prescribed medications and dietary restrictions. Discontinuation of therapy in CKD can be dangerous., as it can lead to rapid worsening of kidney function leading to earlier requirement for initiation of dialysis / kidney transplantation.

Myth: My serum creatinine level is slightly above normal. But I am perfectly well so there is nothing to worry about.

Fact: Even mild increases in serum creatinine can be a sign of kidney dysfunction and needs further attention. A variety of kidney diseases can damage the kidneys, so the nephrologist should be consulted without delay.

In the next paragraph, let us try to understand the importance of an increased serum creatinine (even a little) as it related to the different stages of CKD.

Early stage of chronic kidney disease is usually asymptomatic, and increased serum creatinine may be the only clue of underlying kidney disease. Serum creatinine level of 1.6 mg/dl means that, over 50% of kidney function is already lost, which is significant. Early detection of CKD and initiation of appropriate therapy at this stage is most rewarding. Treatment under the care of a nephrologist at this stage of chronic kidney disease helps to preserve the remaining kidney function for a longer time.

By the time the serum creatinine level goes up to 5.0 mg/dl, 80% of kidney function has already been lost. This value suggests seriously impaired kidney function. Proper therapy at this stage is beneficial to preserve the remaining kidney function. But it is important to remember that this is a late stage of CKD and an opportunity to get the best treatment outcome has unfortunately been lost.

When serum creatinine level is 10.0 mg/dl, it means that 90% of kidney function has already been lost and this points to end stage kidney disease (ESKD). At this stage of CKD, the opportunity to treat a patient with drug therapy is almost lost. Most of the patients need some form of kidney replacement therapy, such as dialysis (or kidney transplantation) at this stage.

Myth: Dialysis performed once in patients with kidney failure, will subsequently become a permanent need.

Fact: No. There are many factors that dictate whether or not dialysis requirement is permanent or temporary.

Acute kidney failure or acute kidney injury (AKI) is temporary and a reversible type of kidney failure. A few patients with AKI may only require dialysis support for a short period of time. With proper treatment and few dialysis treatment sessions, the kidneys usually recover completely in AKI. Delay in dialysis because of fear of permanent dialysis can be life threatening.

CKD is a progressive and irreversible type of kidney failure. Advanced stage of chronic kidney disease (End Stage Kidney Disease) requires regular and lifelong dialysis support or kidney transplantation.

Myth: Dialysis cures kidney failure.

Fact: No, dialysis does not cure kidney failure. Dialysis is otherwise known as kidney 'replacement' therapy. It is an effective and life saving treatment in kidney failure, which removes waste products, excess fluids and corrects electrolytes as well as acid base disturbances. If such substances accumulated in an individual, it can lead to death. Dialysis carries out the function that kidney is no longer capable of doing. Dialysis helps in prolonging survival in patients with severe kidney failure.

Myth: In kidney transplantation males and females cannot donate their kidney to the opposite sex.

Fact: Males and females can donate their kidney to the opposite gender as the structure as well as the functions of the kidneys are similar in both genders.

Myth: Now that my blood pressure is normal, I don't need to take my antihypertensive pills anymore. I feel better if I don't take antihypertensive pills, so why should I take them?

Fact: Many patients with high blood pressure discontinue their medications after the blood pressure is under controlled levels, as they don't have any symptoms and/ or they feel that they are better without antihypertensive medicines. However, uncontrolled hypertension is a silent killer which in the long run can lead to serious problems like heart attacks, kidney failure and strokes. In order, to protect the vital organs of the body, it is essential to continue taking regularly prescribed medications and control blood pressure even in the absence of symptoms.

Myth: Only males have kidneys which are located in a sac between the legs.

Fact: In males as well as in females, kidneys are located in upper and posterior part of abdomen with same size, shape and functions. In males the important reproductive organ, testes is located in a sac between the legs.

Chapter 7

Prevention of Kidney Diseases

Kidney diseases are silent killers. They may cause progressive loss of kidney function leading to kidney failure and ultimately requirement of dialysis or kidney transplant to sustain life. Because of the high cost and potential problems of lack of availability in developing countries, only 5 -10% of patients with kidney failure are fortunate enough to get definitive treatment options such as, dialysis and kidney transplantation, while the rest die without getting any definitive therapy. CKD is very common and has no cure, so prevention is the only option. Early detection and treatment can often keep CKD from getting worse, and can prevent or delay the need for definitive therapy.

How to prevent kidney diseases?

Never ignore your kidneys. Important aspects about care and prevention of kidney diseases are discussed in the following categories.

1. Precautions for healthy individuals.
2. Precautions for individuals with kidney disease.

Precautions for Healthy Person

Seven effective ways to keep the kidney healthy are:

1. Be fit and active

Regular aerobic exercise and daily physical activity maintains normal blood pressure and helps control blood sugar. Such physical activities cut the risk of diabetes and hypertension and thus reduce the risk of CKD.

2. Balanced diet

Eat a healthy diet, full of fresh fruits and vegetables. Decrease intake of refined foods, sugars, fats and meats in the diet. For those above 40 years of age, consuming less salt in the diet may help in the prevention of high blood pressure and kidney stones.

3. Keep your weight in check

Maintain your weight with a balance of healthy food and regular exercise. This can help in preventing diabetes, heart disease and other conditions associated with CKD.

4. Give up smoking and tobacco products

Smoking can lead to atherosclerosis, which reduces blood flow to the kidneys, thus decrease their ability to function at their best. There have also been studies that demonstrate that smoking leads to faster decline in kidney function in those with underlying kidney disease to begin with.

5. Beware of OTCs

Do not overuse over-the-counter (OTC) painkillers on a regular basis. Common drugs such as non-steroidal anti-inflammatory drugs like

Ibuprofen and Naproxen are known to cause kidney damage and subsequent failure particularly, if taken on a regular basis. Consult a doctor to find the best way to control your pain without putting your kidneys at risk.

6. Drink lots of water

Drinking sufficient water (about 3 liters per day) helps to dilute urine, eliminate all the toxic waste from the body and prevent kidney stones.

7. Annual kidney check-up

Kidney diseases are often silent diseases and do not produce any symptoms until they reach an advanced stage. The most powerful and effective but, sadly, underutilized method for early diagnosis and prevention of kidney disease is a regular kidney check-up. Annual kidney check-up is a must for high risk persons who suffer from diabetes, high blood pressure, obesity or have a history of CKD in the family. If you love your kidneys (and, more importantly, yourself), do not forget to get a regular kidney checkup after the age of 40. A simple method for early detection and diagnosis of kidney disease is at least an annual blood pressure measurement, urinalysis and a test to measure creatinine in blood.

Precautions for Kidney Patients

1. Awareness about kidney diseases and early diagnosis

Stay alert and watch for symptoms of kidney disease. Common symptoms of kidney disease are swelling of face and feet, loss of appetite, nausea, vomiting, pallor, weakness, frequent urination,

presence of blood or protein in urine. In the presence of such complaints, it is advisable to consult a doctor and get tests for kidney check up.

2. Precautions in diabetic patient

For all diabetic patients, prevention of kidney disease is particularly essential because diabetes is the leading cause of CKD and kidney failure throughout the world. About 45% of new cases of end-stage kidney disease (ESKD) are due to diabetic kidney disease (DKD). For early diagnosis of diabetic kidney disease, a simple and effective way is at least a tri-monthly measurement of blood pressure and urinalysis to check for the presence of protein or microalbuminuria (MA) by dipstick .This is the best and ideal test for the earliest diagnosis of diabetic nephropathy, which should be done every year. Measure serum creatinine (and estimated glomerular filtration rate, eGFR) to assess kidney function at least once every year.

High blood pressure, presence of protein in the urine, generalized swelling, frequent fluctuations of blood sugar readings, reduction in insulin requirements and appearance of diabetic eye disease (diabetic retinopathy) are important clues to kidney involvement in the presence of diabetes. Beware of these danger signals and consult your doctor immediately.

To prevent DKD, all diabetics should control diabetes meticulously, maintain blood pressure less than 130/80 mmHg (Angiotensin Converting Enzyme inhibitors, ACE-I or Angiotensin Receptor Blockers, ARB are the preferred antihypertensive drugs), reduce the amount of protein in their diet and control lipids.

3. Precautions in hypertensive patients

Hypertension is the second most common cause of CKD. As most people with high blood pressure have no symptoms, many hypertensive patients tend to become non complaint with prescribed treatment or some may even discontinue treatment altogether. Some would discontinue treatment as they feel more comfortable without medicine. But this is dangerous. Uncontrolled hypertension for a prolonged period of time can lead to serious problems like CKD, heart attacks and strokes.

To prevent kidney disease, all hypertensive patients should take regularly prescribed blood pressure medications, get their blood pressures checked regularly and consume a proper diet with appropriate salt restriction. The goal of therapy is to keep the blood pressure less than or equal to 130/80 mmHg. For early diagnosis of kidney damage all hypertensive patients should check urine and blood creatinine every year.

4. Precautions in patients with CKD

CKD is a non-curable disease. But early detection and diagnosis and subsequent dietary restrictions, regular follow up and proper treatment will slow down its progression and may potentially postpone imminent requirement of dialysis or kidney transplantation.

Round the clock proper control of high blood pressure is an effective measure to prevent progression of CKD.

It is highly recommended to keep blood pressure 130/80 mm Hg or below. The best way to attain good control is to monitor the blood pressure regularly at home and maintain a chart, which would immensely help the doctor in adjusting the blood pressure medications accordingly.

In patients with CKD, factors such as hypotension, dehydration, urinary tract obstruction, sepsis, nephrotoxic drugs etc. need to be promptly identified. Prompt management of these factors may lead to maintenance of stable kidney function, and at times, even improvement in kidney function.

5. Early diagnosis and treatment of polycystic kidney disease

Autosomal dominant polycystic kidney disease (ADPKD) is a common and serious hereditary disorder of the kidneys, accounting for 6-8% of patients on dialysis. An adult with a family history of polycystic kidney disease is at a high risk and should be considered for screening by an ultrasound examination for early diagnosis of this disease. PKD has no cure but measures such as controlling high blood pressure, treatment of urinary tract infections, dietary restrictions and supportive treatment help to control symptoms, prevent complications and slow down the rate of decline in kidney function.

6. Early diagnosis and treatment of urinary tract infection (UTI) in children

Urinary tract infection (UTI) should be suspected whenever a child gets unexplained fever, frequent urination, painful burning urination, poor appetite or poor weight gain.

It is important to remember that each bout of UTI, especially with fever carries the potential risk of damage to the kidney, particularly if diagnosed or treated late and inappropriately. Such damage includes scarring of the kidneys, poor kidney growth, high blood pressure and kidney failure later in life. For this reason, it is imperative that UTIs in children are diagnosed early so that appropriate treatment can be rendered immediately; it is also important that when children present with UTIs, identification of predisposing abnormalities (congenital and/ or structural/ anatomic) or other risk factors need to be carried out rather expedetiously. Vesicoureteric reflux (VUR) is the most common predisposing cause present in about 50% of UTIs during childhood. Close monitoring and follow up is mandatory particularly in affected children with UTI.

7. Recurrent urinary tract infections (UTI) in adults

Patients with recurrent UTI or inadequate response to appropriate antibiotic therapy should be evaluated for underlying predisposing factors. Certain underlying causes (e.g. urinary tract obstruction, stone disease etc) carry the risk of permanent damage to the kidney, if it goes untreated. Therefore, early diagnosis and identification of underlying causes is essential.

8. Proper management of benign prostatic hypertrophy (BPH)

Many elderly males with benign prostatic hypertrophy (BPH) neglect their symptoms for a long period of time, because of the misconception that it is normal to have increased frequency of urination or dribbling of urine as they are part of the normal aging process. Untreated BPH can cause permanent damage to the kidneys as well. Proper follow up and timely treatment will help to preserve remaining kidney function at the time of diagnosis.

9. Do not ignore hypertension at young age

Hypertension at a young age is uncommon and almost always requires an exhaustive search for the underlying cause. Kidney diseases are among the most common causes of severe hypertension in the young. Therefore, in young individuals with hypertension, prompt evaluation is mandatory for early detection and diagnosis of kidney disease to prevent progression that may lead to more permanent damage.

10. Early treatment of acute kidney failure/ acute kidney injury (AKI)

Important causes of acute kidney failure (sudden reduction of kidney function) are diarrhea, vomiting, falciparum malaria, hypotension, sepsis, certain drugs (NSAID's) etc. Early and prompt identification of these underlying causes can prevent progression and development of permanent kidney failure.

11. Cautious use of medicine

Be vigilant. Many 'over-the-counter' medications (especially analgesics and pain killers) carry the risk of kidney damage, particularly in the elderly. Such medications are widely advertised, but the likely harmful consequences are rarely disclosed. Avoid the indiscriminate use of over the counter analgesics (pain killers) for headache and generalized body aches. Avoid self medication and unnecessary medications or dietary supplementations. Medications taken under the guidance and supervision of a doctor are usually safe. It is a wrong belief that all natural medicines (Ayurvedic medicines, Chinese herbs etc.) and dietary supplements are harmless. Heavy metals in Ayurvedic medicines have been known to cause irreversible damage to the kidney.

12. Precautions in solitary kidney

Persons with a single kidney can live normal healthy lives.

As in patients with two kidneys, they should keep their blood pressures under control at all times, consume generous amounts of fluids, maintain a healthy diet, avoid excessive salt intake, avoid high-protein diets and avoid injury (e.g., direct trauma) to the solitary kidney. The most important precaution is to have regular medical checkups. One definitely must consult a doctor at least once a year to monitor kidney function by checking the blood pressure, urinalysis and blood tests and undergo a baseline renal ultrasonography, if indicated.

Part 2

Major Kidney Diseases and their Treatment

- Prevention, diagnosis and treatment of kidney failure.

- Basic information about dialysis.

- Basic information about kidney transplantation.

- Important information about major kidney diseases.

- Precaution and selection of diet in patients with chronic kidney disease.

Chapter 8
What is Kidney Failure?

Our kidneys perform several functions in order to maintain balance in our bodies. They filter waste products and excrete them in the urine. They adjust the amounts of water and electrolytes like sodium, potassium and calcium in the body. They also help excrete excess acid or alkali, maintaining acid base balance. A reduction in their ability to perform these tasks is called kidney/renal failure.

How to diagnose kidney failure?

When both kidneys fail, there is a build-up of waste products in the blood, the easiest of which to measure in the laboratory being creatinine and urea. Formulas to estimate kidney function or glomerular filtration rate (GFR) using the serum creatinine are easily accessed on-line or in apps. Importantly, even a slight rise in the serum creatinine reflects a significant decrease in kidney function. A value of just 1.6 mg/dl may indicate over 50% loss of kidney function.

Can failure of one Kidney lead to kidney failure?

No. When only one of two kidneys fails or is removed, overall kidney function may not be significantly affected. The remaining kidney may compensate and take over the workload of both kidneys.

Two major types of kidney failure

Kidney failure may either be acute or chronic in nature.

Acute Kidney Failure

Acute insults to the kidneys may cause a reduction or loss in their function within a short period of time like a few hours to days. This decline in

---

Kidney failure means loss of functions of both kidneys.

---

function was previously called acute renal failure (ARF) but has been recently named Acute Kidney Injury (AKI).

This type of kidney failure is usually temporary. With proper treatment kidney functions return to normal in most patients.

Chronic Kidney Failure

Gradual progressive and irreversible loss of kidney function over several months to years is called chronic kidney disease (CKD), (previously known as chronic renal failure or CRF). Declining kidney function may reach a stage when the kidneys stop working almost completely. This advanced and life-threatening stage of disease is called end stage kidney disease - ESKD (End Stage Renal Disease or ESRD).

When kidney failure is diagnosed, over 50% of kidney function is already lost.

Chapter 9

What is Acute Kidney Injury (AKI)?

In acute kidney injury (previously acute renal failure) reduction or loss of kidney functions occur within a short period (over hours, days or weeks) and is temporary, and usually reversible.

What causes acute kidney injury?

There are many causes of AKI. Common causes include:

1. Reduced blood supply to the kidneys: severe dehydration due to diarrhea, blood loss, burns or fall in blood pressure.

2. Severe infection, serious illness or after a major operation.

3. Sudden blockage of the passage of urine : Kidney stones is the most common cause of urinary tract obstructions.

4. Other causes: Falciparum malaria, leptospirosis, snake bite, certain kidney diseases, pregnancy, complications and side effects of some medications (NSAIDs, aminoglycosides, radio contrast, certain herbal concoctions.

Symptoms of acute kidney injury

In AKI, due to the sudden interruption in kidney function and rapid accumulation of waste products and disturbances in fluid and electrolyte balance, the patient develops early and significant symptoms.

The type of symptoms and their severity differ from patient to patient. These include:

1. Symptoms due to underlying condition (diarrhea, blood loss, fever, chills, etc.) causing kidney failure;

Acute kidney failure is a rapid and usually temporary loss of kidney functions.

---

2. Decreased urine output (urine output may remain normal in a few patients).

3. Swelling of ankles or feet and weight gain due to fluid retention.

4. Loss of appetite, nausea, vomiting, hiccups, fatigue, lethargy and confusion.

5. Severe and life threatening symptoms such as breathlessness, chest pain, convulsions or coma, vomiting of blood and abnormal heart rhythm due to high blood potassium levels.

6. In the early stage of acute kidney failure some patients are symptom-free and the disease is detected incidentally when blood tests are done for other reasons.

Diagnosis of acute kidney injury

Many patients with acute kidney injury have nonspecific symptoms or are asymptomatic. Therefore, in any setting or condition when AKI may develop or in the case of slightest doubt regarding symptoms, one must always suspect and investigate for acute kidney injury.

Diagnosis is confirmed by blood tests (rise in serum creatinine and blood urea), urine output measurements, urinalysis and ultrasound. In patients with acute kidney injury detailed history, examination and different investigations are performed to evaluate causes, complications and progression of the disease.

Treatment of acute kidney injury

In most patients, with proper management acute kidney injury can be reversed.

However delay or improper treatment of severe acute kidney failure can be life-threatening.

> **Symptoms of acute kidney failure are due to both underlying causes and severe kidney problems.**

Major steps for the management of acute kidney injury are:

1. Correction or treatment of the causes of kidney injury.

2. Drug therapy and supportive measures.

3. Dietary advice.

4. Dialysis.

1. Correcting/ treating the causes of kidney injury:

- Identification and treatment of the underlying cause is the most important aspect of management of acute kidney injury.

- Specific treatment of underlying causes such as hypotension, infection, urinary tract obstruction etc. is essential for recovery from kidney failure.

- Such therapy prevents further damage to the kidney and subsequently allows it to recover.

2. Drug therapy and supportive measures:

- The goal is to support the kidneys and to prevent or treat any complications.

- Treatment of infections and avoidance of drugs which are toxic and harmful to the kidney (e.g. NSAIDs).

The use of diuretics such as furosemide help to increase the volume of urine and prevent accumulation of fluid in the body especially the lungs which is a cause of breathlessness.

Supportive therapy: drugs are given which help to correct low or high blood pressure, control nausea and vomiting, control blood potassium, reduce breathlessness and prevent or control convulsions.

In acute kidney failure kidney usually recovers completely with proper treatment.

---

3. Dietary advice

- Proper dietary restriction prevents or reduces symptoms or complications of acute kidney injury.

- Measurement of fluid intake. Daily fluid intake should be planned, keeping in mind urine volume and body fluid status. Usually, restriction of fluid is necessary to prevent edema and complications such as breathlessness.

- Restriction of potassium intake. Avoid potassium-rich food e.g. fruits, fruit juices, dry fruits etc. to prevent high potassium level in blood (hyperkalemia), which is a very serious and life-threatening complication.

- Restriction of salt intake. Salt restriction helps to reduce thirst, edema and complications such as high blood pressure and breathlessness.

- Provision of adequate nutrition and calories.

4. Dialysis

Short-term replacement of the kidney function by dialysis (artificial kidney) may be necessary in a few patients of acute kidney failure until the kidneys recover their functions.

What is dialysis?

Dialysis is the artificial process to replicate the functions of the damaged kidney. It helps to sustain life in people with severe kidney failure. The most important functions of dialysis are to remove wastes, remove excess fluid and correct acidosis and electrolyte disturbances. There are two main types of dialysis : hemodialysis and peritoneal dialysis.

In AKI, the kidneys usually recover completely with proper treatment.

In acute kidney failure with early and proper drug therapy kidney can recover without dialysis.

When is dialysis needed in acute kidney injury?

Dialysis is needed in certain patients with severe forms of acute kidney injury when increasing symptoms and complications occur despite adequate conservative management. Severe fluid overload, uncontrollable hyperkalemia and severe acidosis are the most common indications of dialysis in acute kidney injury.

For how long is dialysis treatment needed in acute kidney injury?

- Certain patients of acute kidney injury need temporary dialysis (hemodialysis or peritoneal dialysis) support till kidney function recovers.

- Patients of acute kidney injury usually recover within 1 - 4 weeks, during which dialysis support may be required.

- Dialysis treatment in AKI is often temporary since the kidneys eventually recover in most cases delaying dialysis because of fear of permanent dialysis can be life-threatening in acute kidney injury.

Prevention of acute kidney injury

- Early treatment of potential causes and frequent check up of kidney function in such patients.

- Prevention of hypotension and its prompt correction.

- Avoidance of nephrotoxic drugs and prompt treatment of infection and reduced urine volume.

Need of dialysis is only for a few days, but delay in dialysis can be life-threatening.

Chapter 10

Chronic Kidney Disease: Causes

Chronic kidney disease (CKD) is a dreaded disease for which medical science has no remedy. CKD is increasing at an alarming rate all over the world. One in ten persons has some form of chronic kidney disease. Rising prevalence of diabetes, hypertension, obesity, smoking, and high cholesterol is major reason for increasing incidences of CKD.

What is chronic kidney disease?

CKD occurs when the kidneys become damaged and gradually unable to perform their functions. With treatment, the kidney function may remain stable, but if not, the damage becomes worse over months to years. The serum creatinine levels rise gradually and the level of kidney function (also called the glomerular filtration rate or GFR) can be calculated from this blood test. The stage CKD can thus be graded as mild, moderate or severe. The presence of albumin in the urine also indicates that kidney damage is present (see tables stage of chronic kidney disease). CKD was previously called Chronic Renal Failure (CRF) but the word failure gives a wrong impression. In early CKD, there is still some degree of renal function and only in the late stages where kidney failure truly occur.

What is end stage kidney disease?

End-stage kidney disease (ESKD) or end-stage renal disease (ESRD) refers to the time when CKD reaches an advanced stage (less than

---

Chronic kidney disease is a gradual, progressive and permanent loss of kidney functions.

10% of normal function). The kidneys may even fail completely and the condition is irreversible.

At this point, conservative management (i.e. medications, diet, lifestyle modifications) is not sufficient to maintain life and renal replacement therapy (dialysis or kidney transplantation) is required.

What causes chronic kidney disease?

A number of conditions can cause permanent damage to the kidneys. But the two main causes of chronic kidney disease are diabetes and high blood pressure. They account for about two third cases of CKD. Important causes of CKD are:

1. Diabetes. Accounting for nearly 35-40 % of all cases, Diabetes is the most common cause of CKD. Roughly every third person with diabetes is at the risk of developing CKD.

2. High blood pressure. Untreated or poorly treated high blood pressure is another leading cause of CKD accounting for nearly 30 % of cases. Furthermore, whatever may be the cause of CKD, high blood pressure will definitely cause further damage to the kidneys.

3. Glomerulonephritis. These disorders which cause inflammation and damage the kidneys are the third in line of ailments that cause CKD.

4. Polycystic kidney disease. This is the most common hereditary cause of CKD characterized by multiple cysts in both kidneys.

5. Other causes: ageing of the kidneys, renal artery stenosis (narrowing), blockage of urine flow by stones or an enlarged prostate, drug-induced and toxin-induced kidney damage, recurrent kidney infection in children and reflux nephropathy.

Two most common causes of chronic kidney disease are diabetes and high blood pressure.

Chapter 11

Chronic Kidney Disease: Symptoms and Diagnosis

In chronic kidney disease (CKD), kidney function gradually declines over months to years. In the early stages of CKD, most patients remain relatively without symptoms as their bodies compensate and get used to the metabolic derangements that develop over time. When the kidney function becomes severely impaired, symptoms due to the accumulation of toxins and fluids start to develop.

What are the symptoms of chronic kidney disease?

Symptoms of CKD vary depending on the severity of the kidney damage. CKD is divided into five stages based on the level of kidney function or glomerular filtration rate (GFR). GFR can be estimated from blood levels of creatinine and is normally greater than 90 ml/min.

CKD Stage 1 (kidney function 90-100 %)

In Stage 1 CKD, the GFR is greater than 90 ml/min/1.73m^2 but there are laboratory abnormalities like protein in the urine; evidence of structural damage to the kidneys on x-ray, ultrasound, MRI, or CT scan; or a family history of polycystic kidney disease. Patients are usually asymptomatic.

CKD Stage 2 (kidney function 60-89%)

In Stage 2 or mild CKD, the GFR is 60 – 89 ml/min/1.73m^2. Patients are usually asymptomatic but some may complain of frequent urination especially at night, high BP, urine abnormalities on urinalysis with normal or slightly high serum creatinine.

**In early stage of CKD most people
do not have any symptoms.**

GFR Categories in CKD			
Stage		Description	Glomerular Filtration Rate (GFR)
At increased risk		With risk factors for CKD (diabetes, high blood pressure, family history, older age, etc)	More than 90
1		Kidney damage (protein in the urine) and normal GFR	More than 90
2		Kidney damage and mildly decreased GFR	60-89
3	3a	Mildly to moderately decreased GFR	45-59
	3b	Moderately to severely decreased GFR	30-44
4		Severely decreased GFR	15-29
5		Kidney failure	Less than 15

National Kidney Foundation Kidney Disease Outcomes Quality Initiative (NKF-K/DOQI) Clinical Practice Guideline for Chronic Kidney Disease

CKD Stage 3 (kidney function 30-59%)

In Stage 3 or moderate CKD, the GFR is 30-59 ml/min/$1.73m^2$. The

Severe uncontrolled high blood pressure at a young age is a common presentation of CKD.

patient may still be asymptomatic or start having mild symptoms. There may be urinary abnormalities present and serum creatinine is elevated.

CKD Stage 4 (kidney function 15-29%)

In Stage 4 CKD, GFR is 15-29 ml/min/1.73m^2. Symptoms may be mild, vague and nonspecific, or very severe, depending on the underlying cause of kidney failure and associated illnesses.

CKD Stage 5 (kidney function less than 15%)

Stage 5 is very severe CKD with GFR of < 15 ml/min/1.73m^2. Also called End Stage Kidney Disease, most patients will need dialysis or kidney transplantation at this stage. Symptoms may vary from moderate to severe, with life-threatening complications.

therapy, sign symptoms of kidney failure increase and most of the patients need dialysis or kidney transplantation.

Common symptoms of kidney diseases

- Loss of appetite, nausea and vomiting.
- Weakness, fatigue and weight loss.
- Swelling (edema) of lower legs.
- Swelling of face or around the eyes especially in the morning.
- High blood pressure, especially if severe, uncontrolled or in young individuals.
- Pallor.
- Sleep problems, lack of concentration and dizziness.
- Itching, muscle cramps or restlessness.
- Flank pains.
- Frequent urination especially at night (nocturia).

CKD is a important cause of low hemoglobin not responding to treatment.

- Bone pains and fractures in adults and retarded growth in children.
- Decreased sexual drive and erectile dysfunction in males and menstrual disturbances in females.

When to suspect CKD in a person suffering from high blood pressure?

In persons with high blood pressure (hypertension) suspect CKD if:

- Age is less than 30 or more than 50 at the time of diagnosis of hypertension.
- Severe hypertension at the time of diagnosis (i.e. more than 200/ 120 mm of Hg).
- Severe uncontrolled high blood pressure even with regular treatment.
- Concomitant visual disturbances.
- Presence of protein in urine.
- Presence of symptoms suggesting CKD such as presence of swelling, loss of appetite, weakness etc.

What are the complications of advanced CKD?

Potential complications of advanced CKD are:

- Severe difficulty in breathing and chest pain due to marked fluid retention in the lungs (pulmonary edema).
- Severe high blood pressure.
- Severe nausea and vomiting.
- Severe weakness.
- Central nervous system complications: confusion, extreme sleepiness, convulsion and coma.

Weakness, loss of appetite, nausea and swelling are common early symptoms of CKD.

- High levels of potassium in the blood (hyperkalemia) which could impair the heart's ability to function and could be life-threatening.
- Pericarditis, an inflammation of the sac-like membrane that envelopes the heart (pericardium).

Diagnosis of CKD

CKD is commonly asymptomatic in early stages. Usually, CKD is initially diagnosed when hypertension is detected, a blood test showing elevated serum creatinine is requested or urine tests positive for albumin. A person must be screened for CKD if he is at high risk for developing kidney damage (diabetic, hypertensive, older age, family history of CKD).

1. Hemoglobin

Hemoglobin levels are usually low. Anemia is due to decreased erythropoietin production by the kidney.

2. Urine test

Albumin or protein in the urine (called albuminuria or proteinuria) is an early sign of CKD. Even small amounts of albumin in the urine, called microalbuminuria, may be the earliest sign of CKD. Since proteinuria can be also due to fever or heavy exercise, it is best to exclude other causes of proteinuria before diagnosing CKD.

3. Serum creatinine, blood urea nitrogen and eGFR

An easy and inexpensive way to measure kidney function is a blood level of creatinine. Together with age and sex, the serum creatinine is used in many formulas to estimate kidney function or glomerular filtration rate (eGFR). Regular monitoring of creatinine helps to assess

---

Three simple tests can save your kidneys. Check blood pressure, urine for protein and eGFR.

---

progression and treatment response in CKD. On the basis of eGFR, CKD is divided into five stages. This staging is useful to recommend additional testing and suggestions for proper management.

4. Ultrasound of the kidney

The ultrasound is a simple, effective and inexpensive test in the diagnosis of CKD. Shrunken kidneys are diagnostic of chronic kidney disease. However, normal or even large kidneys are seen in CKD caused by adult polycystic kidney disease, diabetic nephropathy and amyloidosis. Ultrasound is also helpful to diagnose CKD due to urinary obstruction or kidney stones.

5. Other tests

CKD causes disturbances in different functions of the kidneys. To evaluate these disturbances different tests are performed such as: tests for electrolyte and acid-base balance (sodium, potassium, magnesium, bicarbonate), tests for anemia (hematocrit, ferritin, transferrin saturation, peripheral smear), tests for bone disease (calcium, phosphorus, alkaline phosphatase, parathyroid hormone), other general tests (serum albumin, cholesterol, triglycerides, blood glucose and hemoglobin A1c) and ECG and echocardiography.

When should a patient with CKD contact the doctor?

Patients with CKD should contact the doctor immediately, if he or she develops:

• Rapid unexplained weight gain, marked reduction in urine volume, aggravation of swelling, shortness of breath or difficulty in breathing while lying down in bed.

> **Small and contracted kidneys, seen on ultrasound, are the hallmark sign of chronic kidney disease.**

- Chest pain, very slow or fast heart rate.

- Fever, severe diarrhea, severe loss of appetite, severe vomiting, blood in vomiting or unexplained weight loss.

- Severe muscle weakness of recent origin.

- Development of confusion, drowsiness or convulsion.

- Recent worsening of well controlled high blood pressure.

- Red urine or excessive bleeding.

Chapter 12

Chronic Kidney Disease: Treatment

The three treatment options for CKD are medical management, dialysis or transplant.

- All patients with CKD are treated initially by medical management (medicine, dietary advice and monitoring).
- Severe damage in CKD (ESKD) requires kidney replacement by dialysis or transplant.

Medical Management

Why is medical management very important in CKD?

There is no cure for CKD. Advanced CKD needs dialysis or kidney transplant to maintain life. Because of the high cost and problems of availability, in India only 5 -10% of kidney patients get treatment like dialysis and kidney transplant, while the rest die without getting any definitive therapy. Therefore, early detection and meticulous conservative medical management is the only feasible and less expensive way to manage CKD and delay the need for dialysis or transplant.

Why do many people with CKD fail to take benefit of medical management in CKD?

Initiation of proper therapy at early stages of CKD is most rewarding. Most patients are asymptomatic or feel very well with proper therapy in early stages. Because of the absence of symptoms many patients and their families fail to recognize the seriousness of the disease and discontinue medicine and dietary restrictions. Discontinuation of therapy may lead to rapid worsening of kidney function requiring expensive dialysis or kidney transplantation.

In CKD with early medical management patients can live a long life.

In CKD with early medical management patients can live a long life.

What are the goals of medical management in CKD?

CKD is a progressively deteriorating condition with no cure. The aims of medical management are to:

1. Slow down the progression of the disease.
2. Treat underlying causes and contributing factors.
3. Relieve symptoms and treat complications of the disease.
4. Reduce the risk of developing cardiovascular disease.
5. Delay the need for dialysis or transplant.

What are the treatment strategies in different stages of CKD?

Treatment strategies and recommended actions in different stages of chronic kidney disease are summarized in this table.

Stage	Recommended Action
All Stages	• Regular follow up and monitoring • Life style changes and general measures:
1	• Diagnose/treat to slow down the progression • Educate patients on disease management • Treat comorbid conditions, cardiovascular disease risk reduction
2	• Estimate progression; treat co-morbid conditions
3	• Evaluate/treat complications; refer to nephrologist
4	• Educate patients on kidney replacement options Prepare for kidney replacement therapy
5	• Kidney replacement by dialysis or transplant

**Chronic kidney disease is not curable,
but early treatment is most rewarding.**

Nine Steps of Action Plan in Medical Management of CKD

1. Management of Primary Etiology

Identifying and treating these underlying primary conditions may help prevent, delay or reverse the progression of CKD.

- Diabetes mellitus and hypertension.

- Urinary tract infection or obstruction.

- Glomerulonephritis, renovascular disease, analgesic nephropathy etc.

2. Strategies to Slow Down the Progression of CKD

Your doctor may prescribe important and effective measures to slow down the progression of CKD such as:

- Strict blood pressure control and ACE inhibitor or angiotensin II receptor–blocker therapy.

- Protein restriction.

- Lipid lowering therapy.

- Correction of anemia.

3. Supportive and Symptomatic Treatment

- Water pill (diuretics) to increase volume of urine and reduce swelling.

- Drugs to control nausea, vomiting and gastric discomforts.

- Supplementation of calcium, phosphate binders, active form of Vitamin D and other drugs to prevent and correct CKD related bone disease.

- Correction of low hemoglobin (anemia) with iron, vitamins and erythropoietin injections.

- Prevention of cardiovascular events. Start daily aspirin advised unless contraindicated.

**In CKD treatment of underlying causes
delay the progression of CKD.**

---

4. Management of Reversible Factors

Search and treat reversible factors that may have aggravated or exacerbated the degree of kidney failure. By correction of reversible factors kidney failure may improve, and kidney function may return to stable base level of function. The common reversible causes are:

- Volume depletion.
- Kidney failure due to drugs (non steroidal anti-inflammatory drugs or NSAIDs, contrast agents, aminoglycosides antibiotics).
- Infection and congestive heart failure.

5. Identify and Treat Complications of CKD

Complications of CKD require early diagnosis and immediate treatment. The common complications which need attention are severe fluid overload, high potassium level in blood (potassium > 6.0 mEq/L), and severe ill effects of advanced kidney failure on heart, brain and lungs.

6. Life Style Modification and General Measures

These measures are important in reducing overall risk:

- Stop smoking.
- Maintain healthy weight, exercise regularly and remain physically active on a regular basis.
- Limit alcohol intake.
- Follow a healthy eating plan and reduce dietary salt intake.
- Medications should be taken as directed by the doctor. They may be adjusted according to the severity of the kidney damage.
- Regular follow up and treatment as directed by a nephrologist.

> **Treatment of infection and volume depletion is most rewarding in chronic kidney disease.**

7. Dietary Restrictions

Depending on the type and severity of kidney disease, dietary restrictions are needed in CKD (discussed in detail in Chapter 25).

- **Salt (sodium):** To control high blood pressure and swelling, salt restriction is advised. Salt restriction includes: not adding salt to foods at the table and avoiding salt rich food such as fast food, papad, pickles and minimizing the use of most canned foods.

- **Fluid intake:** Decreased urine volume in CKD patients can cause swelling and in severe cases even breathlessness. Therefore, fluid restriction is advised for all CKD patients with swelling.

- **Potassium** Blood potassium levels usually rise in CKD patients. This can have life-threatening effects on the heart activity. To prevent this, intake of potassium-rich foods (such as dry fruit, coconut water, potatoes, oranges, bananas, tomatoes etc.) should be restricted as advised by a doctor.

- **Protein:** Patients with CKD should avoid high-protein diets which may accelerate the rate of kidney damage.

8. Preparation for Kidney Replacement Therapy

- Protect veins of the non-dominant forearm as soon as CKD is diagnosed.

- Use of the veins of this arm should be avoided for blood collection or IV infusions.

- As kidney function deteriorates and ESKD approaches, dialysis or transplantation will be indicated. A nephrologist will discuss further treatment options with patients and their families, depending on the medical needs of the patient as well as personal preference. Dialysis modalities include hemodialysis or peritoneal dialysis.

In CKD dietary restrictions may delay the progression and prevent complications.

- If hemodialysis is preferred, patients and their families should be educated and advised to have an AV fistula created – preferably 6 to 12 months prior to the anticipated need for initiating hemodialysis.

In CKD, dietary restrictions may delay the progression and prevent complications.

- A CKD patient may also qualify for pre-emptive kidney transplantation. Here, the patient receives a kidney transplant form a live donor prior to the initiation of dialysis.

- Administration of Hepatitis B vaccination in the early stage of CKD reduces risk of Hepatitis B infection during dialysis or kidney transplantation. Four double doses of recombinant Hepatitis B vaccine at 0, 1, 2 & 6 months should be given, intramuscularly in the deltoid region.

9. Referral to a Nephrologist

A person with CKD needs early referral to a nephrologist and pre-dialysis education to decrease morbidity and mortality. Early referral reduces the rate of progression to ESKD and may delay the need to initiate kidney (renal) replacement therapy.

Which is the most important treatment to prevent or delay the progression of CKD?

Whatever the underlying cause of CKD, strict control of blood pressure is the most important treatment to prevent or delay the progression of CKD. Uncontrolled blood pressure leads to rapid worsening of CKD and complications such as heart attack and stroke.

Which drugs are used to control high blood pressure?

The nephrologist or physician will select appropriate agents to control

---

In CKD protect veins of non-dominant forearm by avoiding blood collection or IV infusions.

Most vital treatment to protect the kidney.

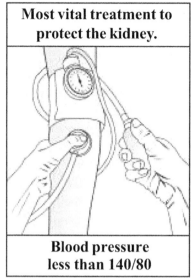

Blood pressure less than 140/80

high blood pressure. The most common drugs used are angiotensin converting enzyme (ACE) inhibitors, angiotensin receptor blockers (ARBs), calcium channel blockers, beta blockers and diuretics.

ACE inhibitors and ARBs are recommended as first line therapy to reduce blood pressure and also helps by slowing the progression of kidney damage, thereby, protecting the kidneys.

What is the goal of blood pressure control in CKD?

It is recommended to keep blood pressure below 130/ 80 mmHg.

Which is the best method to assess and monitor blood pressure control in CKD?

Periodic visits to a doctor help to know the blood pressure status. But buying a blood pressure instrument and using it regularly at home may be helpful to assess and monitor blood pressure control in CKD. Maintaining a chart of blood pressure recordings may help , the doctor adjust drug dosages and times of administration.

How do diuretic drugs help CKD patients?

Doctors may prescribe diuretic which are medicines that help to increase the volume of urine and reduce swelling and breathlessness in some patients. It is important to remember that these medicines may increase the volume of urine but do not improve the function of the kidney.

Why does anemia occur in CKD and how is it treated?

When kidneys are functioning properly, they produce a hormone called erythropoietin, which stimulates the bone marrow to produce red blood cells. In CKD with reduction of kidney function, erythropoietin production also decreases, leading to anemia.

Iron tablets, vitamins and, at times, intravenous iron injections are the first steps to treat anemia due to CKD. Severe anemia, or anemia not responding to drug therapy, needs injections of synthetic erythropoietin, which help bone marrow to produce oxygen-carrying red blood cells. Erythropoietin injections are safe, effective and the preferred method of treating anemia due to CKD. Transfusion of blood is quick and effective to correct anemia in an emergency but is not the preferred method due to the risk of infection and allergic reactions.

Why does anemia in CKD need treatment?

Red blood cells carry oxygen from lungs to all parts of the body. Anemia (low hemoglobin) in CKD leads to weakness, fatigue, poor exercise capacity, breathlessness, rapid heartbeat, loss of concentration, intolerance to cold and chest pain and therefore, this needs early and proper treatment.

> **The most important treatment to delay the progression of CKD is strict control of blood pressure (less than 130/80).**

Dialysis is a procedure by which waste products and excess water that accumulate in renal failure are removed from the body artificially. It is a life-saving technique for patients with End Stage Kidney Disease (ESKD) or Acute Kidney Injury.

How does dialysis help people with severe kidney failure?

Dialysis helps the body by performing the following functions of failed kidneys:

- Purification of blood by removal of waste products such as creatinine, urea etc.

- Removal of excess fluid and maintenance of the right amount of water in the body.

- Correction of electrolyte and acid-base balance disturbances.

However, dialytic therapy cannot replace all the functions of a normal kidney such as production of the hormone erythropoietin needed to maintain hemoglobin levels.

When is dialysis needed?

When the kidney function is reduced by 85-90% from the normal (ESKD) waste products and fluids build up in the body. The accumulation of toxins such as creatinine and other nitrogenous waste products leads to symptoms such as nausea, vomiting, fatigue, swelling and breathlessness. These are collectively termed as uremia. At this point, medical management becomes inadequate and the patient will need to start dialysis.

Dialysis is a prompt and effective treatment modality in symptomatic patients with severe kidney failure.

Can dialysis cure chronic kidney disease?

No. Chronic kidney disease is irreversible and once a patient reaches Stage 5 (ESKD), lifelong dialysis treatments will be needed unless successful kidney transplantation is performed. On the other hand, a patient with AKI may need dialysis support only for a short period until kidney function recovers.

What are the types of dialysis?

There are two main types of dialysis : hemodialysis and peritoneal dialysis.

Hemodialysis: In hemodialysis (HD), waste products and excess fluids are removed from the blood by passing the blood through a special filter or artificial kidney called a dialyzer, aided by a dialysis machine.

Peritoneal dialysis: In peritoneal dialysis (PD), a soft tube or catheter is inserted through the skin, into the abdominal cavity and dialysis solution is infused into the abdominal cavity to remove waste products and excess fluid from the body. This is done at home, usually without a machine.

Which factors determine selection of dialysis modality in ESKD patients?

Hemodialysis and peritoneal dialysis both are effective modalities in ESKD patients. No single dialysis modality is best suited for all patients. After considering advantages and disadvantages of each dialysis modality, selection of HD or PD is made jointly by the patient, family members and the nephrologist. Major factors determining this selection are cost of therapy, age, comorbid conditions, distance of hemodialysis center, educational status, physician bias and the patient's preferences and lifestyle. Because of low cost and easy availability, hemodialysis is preferred by a large number of patients in India.

Dialysis can not cure kidney failure, but helps patients to live comfortably in spite of kidney failure.

Do dialysis patients need to restrict their diet?

Yes. Common dietary recommendations for dialysis patients are restriction of sodium, potassium, phosphorus and fluid intake. Dialysis patients must follow these dietary advices but dietary restrictions are reduced after dialysis is initiated in CKD. Most patients on dialysis are advised to take more protein compared to their pre-dialysis prescriptions, with adequate calories, water-soluble vitamins and minerals. It is advisable that patients on dialysis consult a dietitian to adequately plan their diets.

What is "dry weight"?

In patients undergoing dialysis, the "dry weight" is the weight of the patient after all excess fluid is removed by dialysis. The "dry weight" may need to be adjusted from time to time as the actual weight of the patient may change. This is also known as the edema-free weight, the patient has no lung congestion and the hemodynamic status is not compromised (BP is not low nor do they have any symptoms).

Hemodialysis

In hemodialysis, blood is purified with the help of dialysis machine and dialyzer.

How is hemodialysis done?

Most of the time, hemodialysis is performed in hospitals or free standing dialysis centers, under the care of doctors, nurses and dialysis technicians.

- The dialysis machine pumps blood from the body to the dialyzer through flexible blood tubings. Heparin infusion or continuous saline flushing is done to prevent clotting of blood.

Even after starting dialysis, dietary restrictions must be continued.

- The dialyzer (artificial kidney) is a special filter through which blood flows which removes extra fluids and waste products. Dialyzer purifies blood with the help of special solution called dialysate which is prepared by a dialysis machine.
- Once the blood is cleaned, the machine sends it back to the body.
- Hemodialysis is carried out usually three times per week and each session lasts for about four hours.

How is the blood withdrawn for purification and returned back to the body in the process of hemodialysis?

The three most common types of vascular access for hemodialysis are central venous catheters, native arteriovenous (AV) fistulas and synthetic grafts.

Vascular Access for Hemodialysis		
Right subclavian vein	Right jugular vein	Left femoral vein

1. Central Venous Catheter

- As soon as the decision to start immediate hemodialysis is made, a vascular access or central venous catheter has to be inserted. The vascular access will allow the blood of the patient to leave the body and be brought to the artificial kidney or dialyzer to be cleaned or filtered.

- This method of vascular access is ideal for short-term use until a fistula or graft is ready.

- A catheter is inserted into a large vein in either the neck, chest, or leg near the groin (internal jugular, subclavian and femoral veins respectively). With this catheter more than 300 ml/min blood can be withdrawn for dialysis.

- Catheters are flexible, hollow tubes with two lumens. Blood leaves the patient's body passing through one lumen, enters the dialysis circuit, and is returned to the body via the other lumen.

- Venous catheters are immediate but temporary accesses for hemodialysis especially on emergency cases.

- Two types of venous catheters are available, tunnelled (usable for months) and non-tunnelled (usable for weeks).

2. AV Fistula

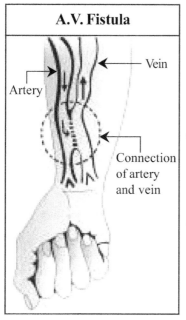

A.V. Fistula

Vein

Artery

Connection of artery and vein

- The arteriovenous or AV fistula is the most common and the best method of vascular access for long term hemodialysis because it lasts longer, & is less likely to get clotted or inflected.

- An AV fistula is created in the forearm near the wrist by surgically connecting or apposing the radial artery to the cephalic vein.

- Since blood flow and pressure is higher in the artery than the vein, blood flows from the former to the latter. After a few weeks or months, the vein dilates and its walls thickens.

Such maturation of the AV fistula takes time, hence, it cannot be used for hemodialysis immediately after its construction.

- For hemodialysis two large-bore needles are inserted into the fistula, one to carry blood to the dialyzer and the other to return the cleansed blood to the body.
- AV fistula lasts for many years if maintained well. All usual daily activities can be easily performed with the hand having AV fistula.

Why does AV fistula need special care?

- Life of a patient with CKD- ESKD depends on regular and adequate hemodialysis. The AV fistula is the permanent vascular access essential for chronic hemodialysis and is also called the lifeline for the patient on maintenance hemodialysis. Special care of AV fistula ensures adequate blood delivery for a long period.
- Large amount of blood with high pressure flows in the veins of AV fistula. Accidental injury to such dilated veins can lead to profuse bleeding, and sudden loss of blood in large volume can be life threatening. So special care is mandatory to protect veins of AV fistula.

Taking Care of AV Fistula

Proper regular care and protection of AV fistula ensures adequate blood delivery for years. Important precautions to keep a fistula healthy and working for longer period are as follows:

1. Prevent infection

Always keep the site of the fistula clean by washing the vascular access arm daily and before each dialysis treatment. It is also important to observe aseptic technique during cannulation and throughout the dialysis process.

AV fistula is the "lifeline" in patients of CKD, without which long term hemodialysis is not possible.

---

2. Protecting the AV fistula

- Use access site only for dialysis. Do not let anyone give intravenous injections, draw blood or measure blood pressure on the arm with the AV fistula.

- Avoid injury to AV fistula. Don't wear jewelry, tight clothes or -a wrist watches on the vascular access arm. Accidental injury to AV fistula can lead to sudden profuse bleeding, which can be life-threatening.

- To control bleeding, immediately apply firm pressure at the site of the bleeding with the other hand or with a tight bandage. After the bleeding is controlled, contact your doctor. Instead of making efforts to control the loss of blood, rushing to hospital for help is unwise and dangerous.

- Do not lift heavy items with the accessed arm and avoid pressure on it. Be careful; do not sleep on the arm with the A V fistula.

3. Ensure proper functioning of AV fistula

Blood flow through the AV fistula should be checked regularly by feeling the vibration (also called a thrill) three times a day (before breakfast, lunch and dinner). If the vibration is absent, your doctor or dialysis center staff should be immediately contacted. A blood clot may have formed inside the fistula and early detection and timely intervention to dissolve or remove the clot may salvage the AV fistula.

- Low blood pressure carries the risk of failure of AV fistula, and therefore, should be prevented.

4. Regular exercise

Regular exercise of AV fistula can lead to its maturation. Even after

> **To ensure adequate blood delivery and effective long term hemodialysis, special care of AV fistula is most essential.**

initiating hemodialysis, regular exercise of access arm helps to strengthen the AV fistula.

3. Graft

- An arteriovenous graft is another form of long term dialysis access, which can be used when persons do not have satisfactory veins for an AV fistula or have a failed AV fistula.

- In graft method, an artery is surgically connected to a vein with a short piece of synthetic soft tube which is implanted under the skin. Needles are inserted in this graft during dialysis treatment.

- Compared to an AV fistula, AV grafts are at a high risk to develop clotting, infection, and usually do not last as long as a fistula.

What are the functions of hemodialysis machine?

- The machine prepares special dialysis solution (dialysate), which is delivered to the dialyzer for cleaning of the blood.

- The machine meticulously adjusts and monitors concentration of electrolytes, temperature, volume and pressure of delivered dialysate, which are modified as per the patient's need. Dialysis solution removes unwanted waste products and extra water from the body through dialyzer.

- For the safety of the patient, the machine has various safety devices and alarms such as for detection of blood leakage from the dialyzer or the presence of air in blood circuit.

- Computerized models of hemodialysis machine with display of various parameters on front screen and different alarms provide convenience, accuracy and safety to perform and monitor dialysis treatment.

The hemodialysis machine, with the help of dialyzer, filters blood and maintains fluid, electrolyte and acid base balance.

What is the structure of the dialyzer and how does it purify blood?

Structure of dialyzer

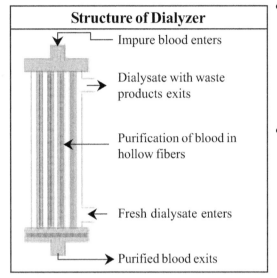

Structure of Dialyzer

Impure blood enters

Dialysate with waste products exits

Purification of blood in hollow fibers

Fresh dialysate enters

Purified blood exits

- In the process of hemodialysis, dialyzer (artificial kidney) is a filter where purification of blood occurs.

- Dialyzer is about 20 centimeter long and 5 centimeter wide clear plastic cylinder which contains thousands of tube-like hollow fibers composed of synthetic semi-permeable membrane.

- These hollow fibers are connected with each other at upper and lower end of the cylinder and form the "blood compartment." Blood enters in the "blood compartment" of hollow fibers from the opening or blood port from one end and exits from the other end after purification.

- Dialysis solution enters from one end of dialyzer, flows around the outside of the fibers ("dialysate compartment") and exits from the other end.

Purification of blood in dialyzer

In hemodialysis, blood flows out from the patient through the vascular access and blood tubings into one end of the dialyzer where it is distributed into thousands of capillary-like hollow fibers. The dialysis solution enters from another port and flows around these fibers in the "dialysate compartment" of the dialyzer.

Process of Hemodialysis

Impure blood enters

Dialysate with impurities

Dialyzer

Dialysate enters

Impure blood from body

Purified blood exits

Blood pump

AV fistula

Purified blood returns

- Every minute, about 300 ml of blood and 600 ml of dialysis solution continuously flow in opposite directions within the dialyzer. The semi-permeable membrane of the hollow fibers which separates the blood and the dialysate allows removal of waste products and excess fluid from the blood to the dialysate compartment.

- Blood exits from the other end of dialyzer after purification. Dialysis solution with toxic substances and excess fluid which are removed from the blood exits from the end of dialyzer from which blood enters.

- In hemodialysis, the blood volume of the patient circulates and passes through the dialyzer about twelve times. After four hours of treatment, blood urea and serum creatinine levels are reduced substantially, excess fluids are removed and electrolyte levels are corrected.

What is dialysate and its function in hemodialysis?

- The dialysate (dialysis solution) is the special fluid used in hemodialysis to remove waste and extra fluid from the blood.

- The composition of the standard dialysate resembles normal extracellular fluid, but depending on the need of the patient, its composition can be modified.

- The dialysate is prepared by manufacturer by mixing about 30 parts of highly purified water with one part of dialysate concentrate.

- The dialysate concentrate is a special fluid that is commercially available, which contains electrolytes, minerals and bicarbonate.

- The water used to make the dialysate is purified sequentially by a sand filter, a charcoal filter, water softener, reverse osmosis, deionization and ultraviolet filtration. The product of these processes is water that is essentially free of dust, suspended impurities, chemical impurities, minerals, bacteria and endotoxins.

- This careful purification of water and subsequent monitoring of its quality is essential to protect patients from the risk of contaminants in the water. Each patient is exposed to about 150 liters of water during each hemodialysis session.

Where is hemodialysis done?

Hemodialysis is usually done in hospitals or dialysis centers by trained staff under the supervision of a doctor. In a few stable patients, it may be done at home. Home hemodialysis requires proper training of the patient and family members, adequate space and financial resources.

Is hemodialysis painful? What does the patient do during dialysis?

The hemodialysis procedure is not painful. There may be slight pain experience during intravenous needle insertion when the blood tubings are connected to the patient at the start of the procedure. This outpatient requires the patient to go to the hospital or dialysis center thrice a week

---

Changes in dialysate composition helps correct electrolyte imbalance and during the process of hemodialysis.

---

and going home afterwards. During the treatment, patients rest, sleep, read, listen to music or watch television. They may even take light snacks and hot or cold drinks during this time.

What are the common problems during hemodialysis?

Common problems during hemodialysis include low blood pressure (hypotension), nausea, vomiting, muscle cramps, weakness and headache. These adverse events may be avoided by appropriately accessing the hemodynamics and volume status before the dialysis session. Weight gain in between sessions should be monitored, as well as serum electrolytes and hemoglobin levels.

What are the advantages and disadvantages of hemodialysis?

Advantages of hemodialysis:

- Since treatments are done by trained nurses or technicians, patients are subjected to less burden of caring for themselves. Some patients find hemodialysis more comfortable and less stressful than peritoneal dialysis.
- Hemodialysis is faster and more efficient per unit time than peritoneal dialysis.
- Hemodialysis center provides a platform to meet and interact with other patients with similar problems. Such interaction can reduce stress and the patient can enjoy company of fellow patients.
- Hemodialysis is usually done for 4 hours, three times a week. Between treatments, patient may enjoy "free time".
- Patients avoid the risks of peritonitis and exit-site infections.
- In some countries, hemodialysis is less expensive than peritoneal dialysis.

The main advantages of hemodialysis are safety, effectiveness and comfort.

Disadvantages of hemodialysis:

- Inconvenience and time lost for regular travel to the hemodialysis center especially when the latter is located far from home.

- Due to fixed schedule for hemodialysis, the patient has to plan all activities around the treatment schedule.

- Frequent needle pricks and insertion during treatments can be painful. There are some measures like application of topical anesthetics to diminish the pain in some cases.

- Dietary restrictions of fluid, salt, potassium and phosphorous still have to be observed. Patients need to adhere to these limitations .

- There is a risk of contracting blood-borne infections like Hepatitis B and C.

Do's and don'ts for hemodialysis patients

- Patients with ESKD on maintenance hemodialysis need regular treatments, usually thrice weekly. Skipping or missing treatments are deleterious to health.

- Hemodialysis patients have to observe proper dietary restrictions. Fluid, salt, potassium and phosphorous restriction have to be observed. Protein intake should be regulated upon the advice of the doctor or renal dietician. Ideally, weight gain between dialysis should be kept at 2 to 3 kgs (4.4 to 6.6 lbs) only.

- Malnutrition is common in patients on hemodialysis and leads to poorer outcomes. A referral to a dietician with the supervision of the doctor is necessary to maintain enough caloric and protein intake to maintain adequate nutrition.

The main disadvantage of hemodialysis is the need to visit a center three times a week.

- Patients on maintenance hemodialysis may need to be supplemented with water-soluble vitamins like vitamins B and C. They should avoid over-the-counter multivitamins which may not contain some required vitamins, may contain inadequate levels of some required vitamins, or may contain vitamins that may be harmful for CKD patients such as vitamins A, E and K.

- Calcium and vitamin D may be supplemented, depending on blood levels of calcium, phosphorus and parathyroid hormone.

- Lifestyle changes are mandatory. General measures include smoking cessation, maintenance of ideal weight, regular exercise and limitation of alcohol intake.

When should a patient on hemodialysis consult a dialysis nurse or doctor?

The patient on hemodialysis should immediately consult a dialysis nurse or doctor in cases of :

- Bleeding from AV fistula site or catheter site.
- Disappearance or absence of vibration, bruit or thrill in the AV fistula.
- Unexpected weight gain, significant swelling or breathlessness.
- Chest pain, very slow or fast heart rate.
- Development of severe high blood pressure or low blood pressure.
- Confusion, drowsiness, unconsciousness or convulsions.
- Fever, chills, severe vomiting, vomiting of blood or severe weakness.

Peritoneal Dialysis

Peritoneal dialysis (PD) is another form of dialysis modality for the patients with kidney failure. It is widely accepted and effective. It is the most common method of dialysis done at home.

> **In patients with hemodialysis restriction of fluids and salt is essential to control weight gain between two dialysis.**

What is peritoneal dialysis?

- The peritoneum is a thin membrane that lines the inner surface of the abdominal cavity.

- The peritoneal membrane is a natural semi-permeable membrane which allows waste products and toxins in the blood to pass through it.

- Peritoneal dialysis is a process of purification of blood through the peritoneal membrane.

What are the types of peritoneal dialysis?

Types of peritoneal dialysis:

1. Intermittent Peritoneal Dialysis (IPD)
2. Continuous Ambulatory Peritoneal Dialysis (CAPD)
3. Continuous Cycling Peritoneal Dialysis (CCPD)

1. Intermittent Peritoneal Dialysis (IPD)

Intermittent peritoneal dialysis (IPD) is a valuable and effective dialysis option for short term dialysis in hospitalized patients with acute kidney failure, in children and during emergencies or initial treatment of ESKD.

In IPD, a special catheter with multiple holes is inserted into the patient's abdomen through which a special solution called the dialysate is infused into the abdominal cavity or peritoneal space. The dialysate absorbs waste products and excess fluids from the patient's blood. After some time, the fluid is drained and the process is repeated several times in a day.

- IPD lasts for a period of 24- 36 hours and about 30 to 40 liters of dialysate solution is used up during the treatment.

- IPD is repeated at short intervals of 1 -3 days, as per the need of the patient.

CAPD is a type of dialysis that can be carried out by patients at home with specialized fluid.

---

2. Continuous Ambulatory Peritoneal Dialysis (CAPD)

What is CAPD?

CAPD means :

C – Continuous: The process is uninterrupted (treatment without stopping for 24 hours a day, 7 days a week).

A – Ambulatory: The patient can walk around and perform routine activities.

P – Peritoneal: The peritoneal membrane in the abdomen works as a filter.

D – Dialysis: The method of purification of blood.

Continuous Ambulatory Peritoneal Dialysis (CAPD) is a form of dialysis which can be carried out by a person at home without the use of a machine. As CAPD provides convenience and independence it is a popular dialysis modality in many countries.

Process of CAPD :

CAPD catheter: The permanent access for peritoneal dialysis (CAPD catheter) is a soft thin flexible silicon rubber tube with numerous side holes. It is surgically inserted into the patient's abdomen through the abdominal wall, about an inch below and to the side of the navel or belly button. The CAPD catheter is inserted about 10 to 14 days before CAPD starts. The PD catheter is the "life line" of CAPD patients, just as the AV fistula is to a patient on hemodialysis.

Technique of continuous ambulatory peritoneal dialysis (CAPD):

In CAPD, special fluid (dialysate) is infused into the abdominal cavity and is kept there for a period of time, after which it is drained. This process of fill, dwell and drain is called an exchange.

**CAPD must be carried out meticulously
every day at a fixed time with no holidays.**

Fill: Peritoneal dialysis fluid from the sterile PD bag is infused by gravity, through sterile tubings connected to the PD catheter, into the abdominal cavity. Usually, 2 liters of fluid is infused. The bag emptied of PD fluid is rolled up and tucked in the patient's inner wear until the next exchange.

Dwell: The period of time in which PD fluid remains inside the abdominal cavity is called the dwell time. This lasts for about 4 to 6 hours per exchange during the day and 6 to 8 hours at night. The process of cleaning the blood takes place during dwell time. The peritoneal membrane works like a filter allowing waste products, unwanted substances and excess fluid to pass from blood into the PD fluid. The patient is free to walk around during this time (hence the term, ambulatory).

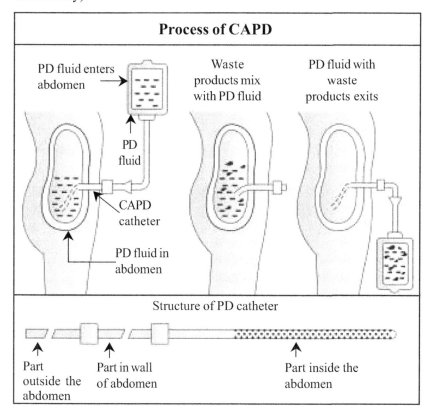

Process of CAPD

PD fluid enters abdomen

Waste products mix with PD fluid

PD fluid with waste products exits

PD fluid

CAPD catheter

PD fluid in abdomen

Structure of PD catheter

Part outside the abdomen

Part in wall of abdomen

Part inside the abdomen

Drain: When the dwell time is completed, the PD fluid is drained into the empty collection bag (which had been rolled up and tucked in the patient's inner clothing). The bag with the drained fluid is weighed and discarded; the weight is recorded. The drained fluid should be clear. Drainage and replacement with fresh solution takes about 30 to 40 minutes. Exchanges may be done from 3 to 5 times during the day and once during the night. Fluid for the night exchange is left in the abdomen overnight and drained in the morning. Strict aseptic precautions should be observed when performing CAPD.

3. APD or Continuous Cycling Peritoneal Dialysis (CCPD):

Automated peritoneal dialysis (APD) or continuous cycling peritoneal dialysis (CCPD) is a form of PD treatment done at home using an automated cycler machine. The machine automatically fills and drains the PD fluid from the abdomen. Each cycle usually lasts for 1-2 hours and exchanges are done 4 to 5 times per treatment. The treatment lasts about 8 to 10 hours, usually at night, while the patient is asleep. In the morning, the machine is disconnected and 2 to 3 liters of PD fluid are usually left in the abdominal cavity. This fluid is drained the following evening before the next treatment is started. APD is advantageous since it allows the patient to go about regular activities during the day. Also, since the PD bag is connected and detached from the catheter only once a day, the procedure is more comfortable and carries less risk of peritonitis. However, APD may be expensive in some countries and can be a rather complex procedure for some patients.

Continuous cycling peritoneal dialysis is carried out at home with an automated cycler machine.

What is PD fluid used in CAPD?

PD fluid (dialysate) is a sterile solution containing minerals and glucose

Continuous Cycling Peritoneal Dialysis is carried out at home with an automated cycler machine.

(dextrose). Glucose in the dialysate allows removal of fluid from the body. Depending on the concentration of glucose, there are three kinds of dialysate available in India and in most areas worldwide (1.5%, 2.5% and 4.5%).The glucose concentration is selected for individual patients depending on the amount of fluid that needs to be removed from the body. Newer PD fluids are available in some countries which contain icodextrin instead of glucose. Icodextrin-containing solutions remove body fluids more slowly and are recommended for diabetic or overweight patients.

CAPD solution bags are available in different volumes ranging from 1000 to 2500 ml.

What are the common problems during CAPD?

The main complications of CAPD involve infections. The most common infection is peritonitis, an infection of the peritoneum Pain in the abdomen, fever, chills and cloudy/turbid outflow of PD fluid (effluent) are common presentations of peritonitis. To avoid peritonitis, CAPD should be done under strict aseptic precautions and constipation should be avoided. The treatment of peritonitis includes broad spectrum antibiotics, culture of the PD effluent (to help select appropriate antibiotics) and, in a few patients, removal of the PD catheter. Infection at the exit site of the PD catheter is another infection that may also develop.

Precautions to avoid infections are of utmost importance in CAPD patients.

Other problems that may occur in CAPD are abdominal distention, weakening of the abdominal muscles causing hernia, fluid overload, scrotal edema, constipation, back pain, poor outflow drainage, leakage of fluid and weight gain.

**Precautions to avoid infections are of
utmost importance in CAPD patients.**

Advantages of CAPD

- Dietary and fluid restrictions are less, compared to hemodialysis treatment.

- More freedom is enjoyed, since PD can be done at home, at work or while travelling. The patient can perform CAPD on his or her own and there is no need for a hemodialysis machine, hemodialysis nurse, technician or family member to help out. Other activities may be done while dialysis is taking place.

- The fixed schedule of hospital or dialysis center visits, travel time and needle pricks associated with hemodialysis are avoided.

- Hypertension and anemia may be better controlled.

- Gentle dialysis with continuous cleaning of blood, so no ups-and-downs or discomfort.

Disadvantages of CAPD

- Infections of the peritoneum (peritonitis) and catheter exit site are common.

- The treatment may be stressful. Patients should perform treatments regularly every day, without fail, meticulously following instructions and strict cleanliness.

- Some patients experience discomfort and changes in appearance due to the permanent external catheter and fluid in the abdomen.

- Weight gain, elevated blood sugar and hypertriglyceridemia may develop due to absorption of sugar (glucose) in the PD solution.

- PD solution bags may be inconvenient to handle and store at home.

What dietary changes are recommended for a patient on CAPD?

- A patient on CAPD requires adequate nutrition and the dietary

---

Main benefits of CAPD are freedom in location, convenience in timings and lesser dietary restrictions.

prescription is slightly different from the diet of patients on hemodialysis.

- The doctor or dietician may recommend increasing protein in the diet to avoid protein malnutrition due to continuous protein loss in peritoneal dialysis.

- Enough calories should be ingested to prevent malnutrition while avoiding excessive weight gain. The PD solution has glucose which adds continuously extra carbohydrate to patient on CAPD.

- Although salt and fluid still have to be restricted, there may be less restriction than for a patient on hemodialysis.

- Dietary potassium and phosphate are restricted.

- Dietary fiber is increased to prevent constipation.

When should a person on CAPD contact the dialysis nurse or doctor?

The patient on CAPD should immediately contact dialysis nurse or doctor when any of the following occurs:

- Pain in abdomen, fever or chills.

- Drainage of cloudy/turbid or bloody PD fluid.

- Pain, pus, redness, swelling or warmth around exit site of CAPD catheter.

- Difficulty in infusion or drainage of PD fluid.

- Constipation

- Unexpected weight gain, significant swelling, breathlessness and development of severe hypertension (suggestive of fluid overload).

- Low blood pressure, weight reduction, cramps and dizziness (suggestive of fluid deficit).

Patients on CAPD must take high protein diet to avoid malnutrition and reduce risk of infection.

Chapter 14

Kidney Transplantation

Kidney transplantation (KT) is the outcome of great advancement in medical science.

Kidney transplantation is the treatment of choice for end-stage kidney disease (ESKD). Successful kidney transplantation may offer better quality of life and longer patient survival compared with dialysis. Life after successful kidney transplantation is almost normal.

Kidney transplantation is discussed in four parts:

1. Pre-Transplant Information
2. Transplant surgery
3. Post Transplant care
4. Deceased donor (Cadaveric) kidney transplant

Pre-Transplant Information

What is kidney transplantation?

Kidney transplantation is a surgical procedure in which a healthy kidney (from a living donor or deceased - cadaver donor) is placed into the body of a person suffering from end-stage kidney disease (recipient).

When is kidney transplant necessary?

Kidney transplantation is necessary for patients who are suffering from ESKD who are on dialysis (hemodialysis or peritoneal dialysis) or who are approaching ESKD but not yet on dialysis (pre-emptive KT).

When is kidney transplant not required in kidney failure?

A patient with acute kidney injury should not undergo KT. Kidney transplantation is also not done in cases where only one kidney fails

---

Discovery of kidney transplantation has been a blessing for patients with chronic kidney failure.

---

and the other kidney is still functioning. Transplantation should only be done if the renal failure is irreversible.

Why is kidney transplant necessary in end-stage kidney disease?

Dialysis replaces some degree of the filtration of waste products of the kidneys. Other functions of the kidneys are not accomplished, some of which are better addressed by transplantation. Hence, kidney transplantation, when a suitable donor is available and when no contraindications are present, offers the best treatment option for complete rehabilitation of a patient with end-stage kidney failure. As kidney transplantation saves lives and enables one to enjoy almost normal life, it is referred to as the "Gift of Life".

What are the advantages of kidney transplantation?

Major benefits of successful KT are:

- Better degree of replacement of renal function and better quality of life: The patient may achieve an almost normal and active lifestyle with more energy, stamina and productivity.

- Freedom from dialysis: Patients avoid the complications, cost, lost time and inconveniences of dialysis treatment.

- Longer life expectancy: Transplant patients have a longer life expectancy than risk-matched patients who remain on dialysis.

- Lesser dietary and fluid restrictions.

- Cost-effectiveness: Although the initial cost of a kidney transplant may be high, the expenses decrease by the second to third year post-transplant and by then, is usually less than that needed for maintenance dialysis treatment.

Successful kidney transplantation is the best treatment option for CKD-ESKD as it offers almost normal life.

- There is a reported improvement in sexual life and a higher chance of fathering a child in males and becoming pregnant in females.

What are the disadvantages of kidney transplantation?

Kidney transplantation offers many benefits but also has disadvantages. These are:

- Risk of major surgery. Kidney transplantation is a major surgical procedure under general anesthesia that has potential risks both during and after the surgery.

- Risk of rejection. There is no 100% guarantee that the body will accept the transplanted kidney. But with the availability of newer and better immunosuppressant drugs, rejections are less likely than they were in the past.

- Regular medication. Transplant patients will need to take immunosuppressive medicines regularly for as long as their donor kidneys are functioning. Discontinuation, missing or not taking the full dosage of immunosuppressant drugs, carries the risk of failure of transplanted kidney due to rejection.

- Risks related to immunosuppressive drugs: Drugs that suppress the immune response and rejection may lead to severe infections . Care to avoid infections and screening for development of some forms of cancer are part of post-transplant care. There are side effects for drugs like high blood pressure, high blood cholesterol and sugar levels.

- Stress. Waiting for a kidney donor before transplant, uncertainty of success of transplant (the transplanted kidney may fail) and fear of

---

Kidney transplantation is not performed in CKD patients with AIDS, cancer and other serious diseases.

---

losing function of the newly transplanted kidney after transplant, is stressful.

- Initial high cost.

What are the contraindications for a kidney transplant?

Kidney transplantation is not recommended if the ESKD patient has:

- A serious active infection
- Active or untreated malignancy
- Severe psychological problems or mental retardation
- Unstable coronary artery disease
- Refractory congestive heart failure
- Severe peripheral vascular disease
- Antibodies against the donor kidney
- Other severe medical problems.

What is the age limit for a kidney transplant recipient?

Although there is no fixed criteria for the age of a kidney transplant recipient, it is usually recommended for persons from 5 to 65 years of age.

What are the likely sources of kidneys for transplantation?

There are three sources of kidneys for transplantation:

- Living related donors: blood relatives of the recipient up to the 4th degree of consanguinity.
- Living non-related donors: like friends, spouses or relatives.
- Deceased (cadaver) donors: from victims of brain death.

Who is the ideal kidney donor?

An identical twin is an ideal kidney donor with the best chances of survival after transplantation.

Kidney donated by family member donors results in most successful kidney transplantation.

Who can donate a kidney?

A healthy person with two kidneys can donate one kidney as long as the blood group, tissue type and tissue crossmatching are compatible with the receipient. Generally, donors should be between the ages of 18 and 65 years.

How does blood group determine the selection of a kidney donor?

Blood group compatibility is important in KT. The recipient and donor must have either the same blood group or compatible groups . Just like in blood transfusions, a donor with blood group O is considered a "universal" donor. (see table below)

Recipient's blood group	Donor's blood group
O	O
A	A or O
B	B or O
AB	AB, A, B or O

Who cannot donate a kidney?

A living donor should be thoroughly evaluated medically and psychologically to ensure that it is safe for him or her to donate a kidney. A person cannot donate kidney if he or she has diabetes mellitus, cancer, HIV, kidney disease, high blood pressure or any major medical or psychiatric illness.

What are the potential risks to a living kidney donor?

A potential donor is evaluated thoroughly to ensure that it is safe for him or her to donate a kidney. With a single kidney, most donors live a

---

**Kidney donation is safe and
saves lives of CKD patients.**

---

normal healthy life. After kidney donation sexual life is not affected. A woman can have children and a male donor can father a child.

Potential risks of kidney donation surgery are the same as those with any other major surgery. Risk of contracting kidney disease in kidney donors is not any higher just because they have only one kidney.

What is paired kidney donation?

Living donor kidney transplantation has several advantages over deceased donor kidney transplantation or dialysis. Many patients with end-stage kidney disease have healthy and willing potential kidney donors but the hurdle is blood group or cross match incompatibility.

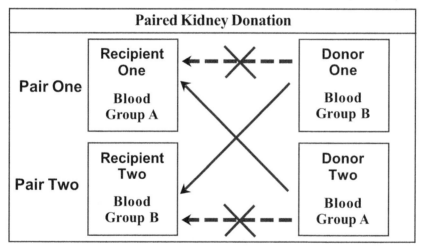

Paired kidney donation (also known as "live donor kidney exchange", "living donor swap" or "kidney swap") is the strategy which allows the exchange of living donor kidneys between two incompatible donor/recipient pairs to create two compatible pairs. This can be done if the second donor is suitable for the first recipient, and the first donor is suitable for the second recipient (as shown above). By exchanging the donated kidneys between the two incompatible pairs, two compatible transplants can be performed.

What is pre-emptive kidney transplant?

Kidney transplantation usually takes place after a variable period of dialysis therapy. Kidney transplantation may be done before the initiation of maintenance dialysis when the renal function is less than 20 ml/min. This is called a pre-emptive KT.

Pre-emptive KT is considered the best option for kidney replacement therapy in medically suitable patients with end stage kidney disease (ESKD) because it not only avoids the risks, cost, and inconvenience of dialysis, but also is associated with better graft survival than transplantation performed after initiating dialysis. Because of its benefits, one is strongly advised to consider a pre-emptive transplantation in ESKD, if a suitable donor is available.

Transplant Surgery

How is a kidney transplanted?

- Before surgery, medical, psychological and social evaluation is done to ensure fitness and safety of both the recipient and the donor (in living-kidney donor transplant). Testing also ensures proper blood group and HLA matching and tissue crossmatching.

- Kidney transplantation is a teamwork of the nephrologists, transplant surgeon, pathologist, anesthesiologist and supporting medical (cardiologist, endocrinologist, etc) and nursing staff as well as transplant coordinators.

- After a thorough explanation of the procedure a careful reading of the consent form, consent of both the recipient and the donor (in living kidney donation) is obtained.

In kidney transplantation, kidney is transplanted in lower abdomen of the recipient without disturbing old kidneys.

Kidney Transplantation

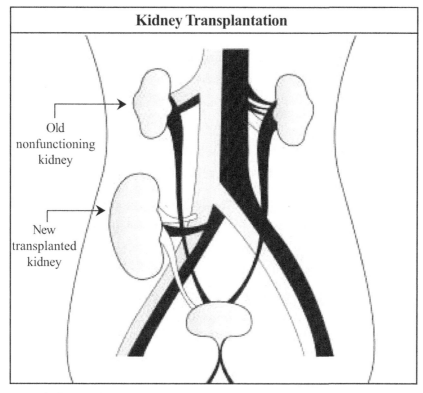

Old nonfunctioning kidney

New transplanted kidney

- In living-kidney donor transplant surgery, both the recipient and the donor are operated on simultaneously.

- This major surgery lasts from three to five hours and is performed under general anesthesia.

- In living-kidney donor transplant surgery, usually the left kidney is removed from the donor either by open surgery or by laparoscopy. After removal, the kidney is washed with a special cold solution and subsequently placed into the right lower (pelvic) part of the abdomen of the recipient.

- In most cases, the old diseased kidneys of the recipient are not removed.

- When the source of kidney is a living donor, the transplanted kidney usually begins functioning immediately. However, when the source of the kidney is a deceased (cadaver) kidney donor, the transplanted kidney may take a few days or weeks to begin functioning. The recipient with delayed functioning transplanted kidney needs dialysis until kidney function becomes adequate.

- After the transplant, the nephrologist supervises the monitoring and medications of the recipient. Living donors should also be screened and monitored regularly for any health issues that may develop.

Post-Transplant Care

What are the likely post-transplant complications?

The common possible complications after transplantation include rejection, infection, medication side effects and post-operative complications. Major considerations in post-transplant care are:

- Post-transplant medications and kidney rejection.
- Precautions to keep the transplanted kidney healthy and to prevent infections.

Post-transplant Medications and Kidney Rejection

How does post-surgical management of kidney transplantation differ from other routine surgery?

In most cases of routine surgery, post-surgical medications and care are needed for about 7-10 days. However, after kidney transplantation, lifelong regular medications and meticulous care are mandatory.

What is kidney rejection?

The immune system of the body is designed to recognize and destroy foreign proteins and antigens like harmful bacteria and viruses. When the recipient's immune system recognizes that the transplanted kidney is not 'its own,' it attacks the transplanted kidney and tries to destroy it.

> **Major post-transplant complications are kidney rejection, infection and side effects of drugs.**

This attack by the body's natural defense on a transplanted kidney is known as rejection. Rejection occurs when the transplanted kidney is not accepted by the body of the transplant recipient.

When does kidney rejection occur and what is its effect?

Rejection of the kidney can occur at any time after the transplant, most commonly in the first six months. The severity of rejection varies from patient to patient. Most rejections are mild and easily treated by proper immunosuppressant therapy. In a few patients however, rejection may be severe not responding to therapy and eventually destroying the kidney.

What medications should a patient take after transplant to prevent rejection?

- Because of the immune system of the body, there is always a risk of rejection of the transplanted kidney.

- If the immune system of the body is suppressed the risk of rejection is decreased. However, the patient becomes prone to life-threatening infections.

- Special drugs are given to patients after kidney transplantation to selectively alter the immune system and prevent rejection, but minimally impair the ability of the patient to fight infections.

Such special drugs are known as immunosuppressant drugs.

At present, the most widely used immunosuppressant drugs are tacrolimus/cyclosporine, mycophenolate mofetil (MMF), sirolimus/everolimus and prednisolone.

How long does the patient need to continue immunosuppressant drugs after kidney transplant?

Immunosuppressant medications have to be given throughout life, for

---

After kidney transplantation lifelong drug therapy is mandatory to prevent kidney rejection.

---

as long as the kidney graft is functioning. In the immediate post transplant period, several drugs are given but their numbers and dosages are gradually reduced over time.

Does the patient need any other medication after kidney transplant?

Yes. After kidney transplant, in addition to immunosuppressant drugs, antihypertensive drugs, calcium, and medications to treat or prevent infection and anti-peptic ulcer medications may be prescribed.

What are the common side effects of immunosuppressant drugs?

Common side effects of immunosuppressant drugs are summarized in the following table.

Drugs	Common side effects
Prednisolone	Weight gain, high blood pressure, gastric irritation, increased appetite, increased risk of diabetes, osteo porosis, cataract
Cyclosporine	High blood pressure, mild tremor, excess hair growth, swelling of gum, increased risk of diabetes, kidney damage
Azathioprine.	Bone marrow suppression, increased risk of infection
MMF	Abdominal pain, nausea, vomiting and diarrhea
Tacrolimus	High blood pressure, diabetes, tremor, headache, kidney damage
Sirolimus/ everolimus	High blood pressure, low blood cell count, diarrhea, acne, joint pain, increased cholesterol, triglycerides

---

If a transplanted kidney fails, initiation of dialysis and a second transplant are two treatment options.

What happens if transplanted kidney fails?

When a transplanted kidney fails, the patient may either undergo a second transplant or undergo dialysis.

Precautions after kidney transplant

Successful kidney transplant provides a new, normal, healthy and independent life. However, the recipient must live a disciplined lifestyle and follow precautions to protect the transplanted kidney and prevent infections. The patient has to be compliant and take prescribed medications regularly and without fail.

General guidelines to keep transplanted kidney healthy

- Never stop taking medication or modify its dosage. Remember that irregularity, modification or discontinuation of medications are some of the most common reasons for transplant failure.

- Always keep a list of medications and maintain adequate stock. Do not take any over-the-counter drugs or herbal therapies.

- Blood pressure, volume of urine, weight and blood sugar (if advised by the doctor) every day.

- Regular follow up with a doctor and laboratory tests as advised, is mandatory.

- Get blood tested in reputed laboratories only. If laboratory reports are not satisfactory, rather than changing the laboratory, it is advisable to consult your doctor at the earliest.

- In an emergency, if you need to consult a doctor who is unaware about your disease, do not fail to inform him that you are a transplant recipient and brief him about the medications.

- There are less dietary restrictions after transplantation. Meals should

---

Keys for success in post-transplant period are regularity, precautions and watchfulness.

---

be taken regularly. One should eat a well-balanced diet with adequate calories and proteins as prescribed. Eat foods low in salt, sugar, and fat and high in fiber to avoid weight gain.

- Water intake should be adequate to avoid dehydration. Patients may require up to more than three liters of water a day.

- Exercise regularly and keep weight under control. Avoid heavy physical activity and contact sports e.g. boxing, football.

- Safe sexual activities can be resumed after about two months, after consulting the doctor.

- Avoid smoking and alcohol intake.

- Stay away from crowded places such as cinemas, shopping malls, public transportation and people who have infections.

- Always wear a face mask in public places and high-risk areas such as construction sites dust-laden environments, excavation sites, caves, animal care settings, farms, gardens, etc.

- Always wash your hands with soap and water before you eat, before preparing or taking medications and after using the bathroom.

- Drink filtered boiled water.

- Eat fresh home-cooked cooked food in clean utensils. Avoid eating meals cooked outside the home and raw, uncooked foods. Avoid raw fruits and vegetables for the first 3 months after transplant.

- Maintain proper cleanliness at home.

- Take good care of teeth by brushing twice a day.

- Do not neglect any cuts, abrasions or scrapes. Promptly clean them with soap and water cover them with clean dressing.

Immediately consulting a doctor and promptly treating any new or unusual problem are mandatory to protect the kidney.

Consult or call the doctor or transplant clinic in case of:

- Fever over 100 F or 37.8 C and flu-like symptoms such as chills, body aches or persistent headache.

- Pain or redness over or around the transplanted kidney.

- Significant decrease in urine output, fluid retention (swelling) or rapid weight gain (more than 1 kg in a day).

- Blood in the urine or burning sensation during urination.

- Cough, breathlessness, vomiting or diarrhea.

- Development of any new or unusual symptoms.

- Immediately contacting the doctor and promptly treating any new or unusual problem are mandatory to protect the kidney.

Why are only a few patients with kidney failure able to get kidney transplants?

A kidney transplant is the most effective and best treatment option for patients with chronic kidney disease - end stage kidney failure. There is a large number of patients who need or wish to obtain a kidney transplant. There are three important reasons for the limited feasibility of the procedure.

1. **Unavailability of kidney:** Only a few patients are lucky to obtain either living (related or non-related) or deceased (cadaveric) kidney donors. Major problems are the limited availability of living donors and the long waiting list for deceased donors.

2. **Cost:** The cost of transplant surgery and the post-transplant lifelong medications is very high. This is a major hurdle for a large number of patients in developing countries.

3. **Lack of facilities:** In many developing countries, facilities for kidney transplantation are not readily or easily available.

The scarcity of kidney donors is a major hurdle which deprives patients from the benefits of a transplant.

Deceased (Cadaveric) Kidney Transplantation

What is deceased kidney transplantation?

Deceased (cadaver) transplantation involves transplanting a healthy kidney from a patient who is "brain dead" into a patient with CKD. The deceased kidney comes from a person who has been declared "brain dead" with the desire to donate organs having been expressed either by the family or by the patient previously, at the event of his/her death.

Why are deceased kidney transplants necessary?

Due to the shortage of living donors, many CKD patients, though keen to have a transplant, have to remain on maintenance dialysis. The only hope for such patients is a kidney from deceased or cadaver donors. The most noble human service is being able to save the lives of others after death by donating organs. A deceased kidney transplant also helps eliminate illegal organ trade and is the most ethical form of kidney donation.

What is "Brain Death"?

"Brain death" is the complete and irreversible cessation (stopping) of all brain functions that leads to death. The diagnosis of "brain death" is made by doctors in hospitalized unconscious patients on ventilator support.

Criteria for diagnosis of brain death are:

1. The patient must be in a state of coma and the cause of the coma (e.g. head trauma, brain hemorrhage etc) is firmly established by history, clinical examination, laboratory testing, and neuroimaging. Certain medications (e.g. sedatives, anticonvulsants, muscle relaxants,

> **In "Brain Death" damage is irreversible with no chances of improvement by any medical or surgical treatment.**

anti-depressants, hypnotics and narcotics), metabolic and endocrine causes can lead to an unconscious state that can mimic brain death. Such causes have to be excluded before confirming the diagnosis of brain death. The doctor should correct low blood pressure, low body temperature and low body oxygen before considering brain death.

2. Persistent deep coma in spite of proper treatment under care of experts for an adequate period to "exclude the possibility of recovery".

3. No spontaneous breathing, patient is on ventilator support.

4. Respiration, blood pressure and blood circulation is maintained with ventilator and other life support devices.

What is the difference between brain death and unconsciousness?

An unconscious patient may or may not need the support of a ventilator and is likely to recover after proper treatment. In a patient with "Brain Death," the brain damage is severe and irreversible and is not expected to recover despite any medical or surgical treatment. In a patient with "Brain Death", as soon as the ventilator is switched off, respiration stops and the heart stops beating. It is important to remember that the patient is already legally dead and removing the ventilator is not the cause of death. Patients with "Brain Death" cannot remain on ventilator support indefinitely, as their heart will stop relatively soon.

Is it possible to donate a kidney after dying?

No. Death occurs after the heart and respiration stop irreversibly and permanently. Like corneal donation, after death, kidney donation is not possible. When the heart stops, the blood supply to the kidney

---

In "Brain Death" the body's respiration and blood circulation are artificially maintained after death.

---

also stops, leading to severe and irreversible damage to the kidney, preventing its use for kidney transplantation.

What are the common causes for "Brain Death?"

Common causes of brain death are head injuries (i.e. falls or vehicular accidents), intracranial brain hemorrhage, brain infarct and brain tumor.

When and how is "Brain Death" diagnosed? Who diagnoses "Brain Death?"

When a deeply comatose patient kept on ventilator and other life supporting devices for an adequate period does not show any improvement on clinical and neurological examination, the possibility of "Brain Death" is considered. Diagnosis of brain death is made by a team of doctors who are not involved in kidney transplantation This team includes the attending physician, neurologist or neurosurgeon, who, after independent examinations of the patient, declare "brain death." By detailed clinical examination, various laboratory tests, special EEG test for brain and other investigations, all possibilities of recovery from brain damage are explored. When no chance of any recovery is confirmed, "brain death" is declared.

What are the contraindications for kidney donation from a patient with "Brain Death?"

Under the following conditions a kidney cannot be accepted from a donor with brain death:

1. A patient with active infections.

2. A patient suffering from HIV or hepatitis B or C.

3. A patient with long standing hypertension, diabetes mellitus, kidney disease or presence of kidney failure.

4. Cancer patient (except brain tumor).

One deceased donor can save the lives of two CKD patients as he donates both his kidneys.

Which other organs can be donated by cadaver donors?

Cadaver donors can donate both kidneys and save lives of two patients. Besides kidney, other organs which can be donated are eye, heart, liver, skin, pancreas etc.

Who comprise the team for deceased kidney transplantation?

For deceased (cadaveric) kidney transplantation proper team work is necessary. The team ncludes:

- Relatives of the deceased kidney donor for legal consent.
- Attending physician of the donor.
- Cadaver transplant coordinator, who explains and helps the relatives of the patient for kidney donation.
- Neurologist who diagnoses the brain death.
- Nephrologist, urologist, transplant surgeon and team.

How is deceased kidney transplantation performed?

These are essential aspects of deceased kidney transplantation.

- A proper diagnosis of brain death is mandatory.
- The donor kidneys should be confirmed to be reasonably healthy and the donor should have no systemic disease that would contraindicate donation.
- Consent to donation should be given by a relative or person who is legally allowed to do so.
- Donor is kept on ventilator and other life-supporting devices to maintain respiration, heart beat and blood pressure until both kidneys are removed from the body.

After kidney transplantation the patient can enjoy a normal and active lifestyle.

- After removal, the kidney is processed properly with a special cold fluid and is preserved in ice.

  One deceased donor can donate both kidneys, so two recipients can be given the gift of life.

- Appropriate recipients are selected from a waiting list of patients following a protocol based on blood group, HLA matching and tissue cross matching compatibility.

- Better outcomes are expected the earlier the harvested kidneys are transplanted. They should ideally be transplanted within 24 hours of harvest. Beyond a certain length of time, they may not be viable for transplantation anymore.

- The surgical procedure on the recipient is the same for both living or deceased kidney donation.

- During the period of time between harvest and transplantation, the donor kidney sustains some damage due to lack of oxygen, lack of blood supply and cold exposure from storage in ice. Because of such injury, the kidney may not function immediately after transplantation and on occasion, short term dialysis support may be necessary while waiting for the donor kidney to recover and regain function.

Is there any payment made given to the donor's family?

None. Giving another person a new lease on life is an invaluable gift. Being a donation, the donor or the donor's family should not expect to receive any payment in exchange for the donated kidney, neither does the recipient need to pay anyone. The joy and satisfaction for this humanitarian gesture should be enough compensation for the donor or the family

---

**Organ donation is a spiritual act.
What can be more sacred than saving a life?**

Chapter 15

Diabetic Kidney Disease

The number of people suffering from diabetes mellitus is increasing all over the world. The impact of a growing number of diabetic patients is an increase in the incidence of diabetic kidney disease, one of the worst complications of diabetes that carries a high mortality.

What is diabetic kidney disease?

Persistent high blood sugar damages small blood vessels of the kidney in long-standing diabetes. This damage initially causes loss of protein in the urine. Subsequently it causes hypertension, swelling and symptoms of gradual damage to the kidney. Finally, progressive deterioration leads to severe kidney failure (ESKD). This diabetes induced kidney problem is known as diabetic kidney disease. Diabetic nephropathy is the medical term used for diabetic kidney disease.

Why is it important to learn about diabetic kidney disease?

- The incidence of diabetes is growing very fast throughout the world.
- Diabetic kidney disease (diabetic nephropathy) is the number one leading cause of chronic kidney disease.
- Diabetes mellitus is responsible for 40-45 % of newly diagnosed patients with end stage kidney disease (ESKD).
- Therapy of ESKD is costly and may be unaffordable for patients in developing countries.
- Early diagnosis and treatment can prevent diabetic kidney disease. In diabetics with established chronic kidney disease, meticulous

---

Diabetes is the most common cause of chronic kidney disease.

---

therapy can postpone the need for dialysis and transplantation significantly.

- There is an increased risk of death from cardiovascular causes in patients with diabetic kidney disease.
- Early diagnosis of diabetic kidney disease is therefore essential in the care of the diabetic patient.

How many diabetics develop diabetic kidney disease?

There are two major types of diabetes mellitus, each with different risks of developing diabetic kidney disease.

Type 1 Diabetes (IDDM - Insulin Dependent Diabetes Mellitus): Type 1 diabetes usually occurs at a young age and insulin is needed to control it. About 30 - 35% of Type 1 diabetics develop diabetic kidney disease.

Type 2 Diabetes (NIDDM - Non Insulin Dependent Diabetes Mellitus): Type 2 diabetes usually occurs in adults and is controlled without insulin in most of the patients. About 10 - 40% of Type 2 diabetics develop diabetic kidney disease. Type 2 diabetes is the number one cause of chronic kidney disease, responsible for more than one of every three new cases.

Which diabetic patient will develop diabetic kidney disease?

It is difficult to predict which diabetic patient will develop diabetic kidney disease. But major risk factors for its development are:

- Type 1 diabetes with onset before 20 years of age
- Poorly controlled diabetes (higher HbA1c levels)
- Poorly controlled high blood pressure
- Family history of diabetes and chronic kidney disease

Diabetes is the cause of end stage kidney disease in one out of three patients on dialysis therapy.

- Vision problem (diabetic retinopathy) or nerve damage (diabetic neuropathy) due to diabetes

- Presence of protein in urine, obesity, smoking and elevated serum lipids

When does diabetic kidney disease develop in a diabetic patient?

Diabetic kidney disease takes many years to develop, so it rarely occurs in the first 10 years of diabetes. Symptoms of diabetic kidney disease manifest 15 to 20 years after the onset of Type 1 diabetes. If a diabetic person does not develop diabetic kidney disease in the first 25 years, the risk of it ever developing decreases.

When does one suspect diabetic kidney disease in a diabetic patient?

Diabetic kidney disease can be suspected in a diabetic patient in the presence of:

- Foamy urine or the presence of albumin/protein in the urine (seen in early stage).

- High blood pressure or worsening of pre-existing high blood pressure.

- Swelling of the ankles, feet and face; reduced urine volume or weight gain (from accumulation of fluid).

- Decreased requirement of insulin or anti-diabetic medications.

- History of frequent hypoglycemia (low sugar level). Better control of diabetes with the dose of anti-diabetic medications with which diabetes was controlled poorly in the past.

- Diabetes controlled without medicine. Many patients feel proud and

---

Signs of harmful effects of diabetes on kidney are excess protein in urine, high blood pressure and swelling.

happy with sugar control, thinking that diabetes has been cured, but the unfortunate and actual fact is that the person has worsening kidney failure. Anti-diabetic medications have a prolonged effect in patients with kidney failure.

- Symptoms of chronic kidney disease (weakness, fatigue, loss of appetite, nausea, vomiting, itching, pallor and breathlessness), which develop in later stages.

- Elevated values of creatinine and urea in blood tests.

How is diabetic kidney disease diagnosed and which test detects it at the earliest?

The two most important tests used to diagnose diabetic kidney disease are the urine test for protein and the blood test for creatinine (and eGFR). The ideal test to detect diabetic kidney disease at the earliest is a test for microalbuminuria (see below). The next best diagnostic test is the urine test for albumin by standard urine dipstick test, which detects macroalbuminuria. Blood tests for creatinine (and eGFR) reflect kidney function with higher values of serum creatinine indicating more severe renal function and increasing in the later stage of diabetic kidney disease (usually after the development of macroalbuminuria).

What is microalbuminuria and macroalbuminuria?

Albuminuria means the presence of albumin (type of protein) in urine. Microalbuminuria, which indicates the presence of a small amount of protein in urine (urine albumin 30-300 mg/day), cannot be detected by a routine urinalysis. It can only be detected by special tests. Macroalbuminuria, which indicates the presence of a large amount of albumin in the urine (urine albumin > 300 mg/day), can be detected by routinely performed urine dipstick tests.

> **Warning: Frequent reduction of blood sugar or diabetes controlled without medication--suspect diabetic kidney disease.**

Why is the urine test for microalbuminuria the most ideal test for the diagnosis of diabetic kidney disease?

Because the test for microalbuminuria can diagnose diabetic kidney disease at the earliest, it is the most ideal test for the diagnosis. Early diagnosis of diabetic kidney disease in this stage (known as high risk stage or incipient stage) is beneficial for patients because if detected early, diabetic kidney disease can be prevented and reversed with meticulous treatment.

The microalbuminuria test can detect diabetic nephropathy 5 years earlier than standard dipstick urine tests and several years before it becomes dangerous enough to cause symptoms or an elevated serum creatinine value. In addition to the risk to kidney, microalbuminuria independently predicts a high risk of developing cardiovascular complications in diabetic patients.

Early diagnostic ability of the microalbuminuria warns patients about developing the dreaded disease and provides doctors the opportunity to treat such patients more vigorously.

When and how often should a urine test for microalbuminuria be done in diabetics?

In Type 1 diabetes, the test for microalbuminuria should be done 5 years after the onset of diabetes and every year thereafter. In Type 2 diabetes, the test for microalbuminuria should be done at the time of diagnosis and every year thereafter.

How is urine tested for microalbuminuria in diabetics?

For screening of diabetic kidney disease, random urine is tested first by standard urine dipstick test. If protein is absent in this test, a more

Two most important diagnostic tests of diabetic kidney disease are urine test for protein and serum creatinine.

precise urine test is performed to detect microalbuminuria. If urine albumin is present in routine test, there is no need to test for microalbuminuria. To diagnose diabetic nephropathy correctly, two out of three tests for microalbuminuria need to be positive within a three- to six-month period in the absence of a urinary tract infection.

Three most common methods used for the detection of microalbuminuria are:

Spot urine test: This test is performed using a reagent strip or tablet. It is a simple test which can be performed in an office practice and is less expensive. Because this test is less accurate, a positive test using a reagent strip or tablet should be confirmed by a urine albumin to creatinine ratio.

Albumin-to-creatinine ratio: Urinary albumin-to-creatinine ratio (ACR) is the most specific, reliable and accurate method of testing microalbuminuria. ACR estimates 24-hour urine albumin excretion. In an early morning urine sample, albumin-to-creatinine ratio (ACR) between 30-300 mg/g is diagnostic of microalbuminuria (normal value of ACR < 30 mg/g). Because of the problem of availability and cost, the number of diabetic patients in whom diagnosis of microalbuminuria is established by this method is limited in developing countries.

24-hour urine collection for microalbuminuria: Total urine albumin of 30 to 300 mg in a 24 hour urine collection suggests microalbuminuria. Although this is a standard method for the diagnosis of microalbuminuria, it is cumbersome and adds little to prediction or accuracy.

> **Urine test for microalbuminuria is the first and most accurate test for the diagnosis of diabetic kidney disease.**

How does standard urine dipstick test help in the diagnosis of diabetic kidney disease?

The standard urine dipstick test (often reported as "trace" to 4+) is the most widely and routinely used method for detection of protein in urine. In patients with diabetes, the standard urine dipstick test is an easy and quick method to detect macroalbuminuria (urine albumin >300 mg/day). The presence of macroalbuminuria reflects stage 4 - overt diabetic kidney disease.

In the development of diabetic kidney disease, macroalbuminuria follows microalbuminuria (stage 3 - incipient diabetic kidney disease), but usually precedes more severe kidney damage, i.e. nephrotic syndrome, and the rise in serum creatinine due to chronic kidney disease.

While the detection of microalbuminuria identifies the patients with diabetic kidney disease early, its cost and unavailability in developing countries limits its use. In such a scenario, the urine dipstick test to diagnose macroalbuminuria is the next best diagnostic option for diabetic kidney disease.

The urine dipstick test is a simple and cheap method and is readily available even in small centers. It is therefore an ideal and feasible option for the mass screening of diabetic kidney disease. Vigorous management even at this stage of diabetic kidney disease is rewarding and may delay the need for dialysis or kidney transplantation.

How is diabetic kidney disease diagnosed?

Ideal method: Annual screening of diabetic patients by testing the urine for microalbuminuria and testing blood for creatinine (and eGFR).

Annual urine test for microalbuminuria is the best strategy for the early diagnosis of diabetic kidney disease.

Practical method: Three monthly measurements of blood pressure and urine dipstick test; and annual blood test for creatinine (and eGFR) in all diabetic patients. This method of detection of diabetic kidney disease is easily affordable and possible even in small towns of developing countries.

How can diabetic kidney disease be prevented ?

Important tips to prevent diabetic kidney disease include:

- Follow up regularly with the doctor.
- Achieve the best control of blood sugar. Keep HbA1C levels less than 7%.
- Keep blood pressure below 130/80 mmHg. Antihypertensive drugs called angiotensin-converting enzyme (ACE) inhibitors or angiotensin receptor blockers (ARBs) should be used to control hypertension and aid in the reduction of albuminuria.
- Restrict sugar and salt intake and eat a diet low in protein, cholesterol and fat.
- Check kidneys at least once a year by performing a urine test for albumin and blood test for creatinine (and eGFR).
- Other measures: Exercise regularly and maintain ideal weight. Avoid alcohol, smoking, tobacco products and indiscriminate use of painkillers.

Treatment of diabetic kidney disease

- Ensure proper control of diabetes.
- Meticulous control of blood pressure is the most important measure to protect the kidneys. Blood pressure should be measured regularly

---

Urine dipstick test to diagnose macroalbuminuria is the most feasible diagnostic option for developing countries.

and maintained below 130/80 mmHg. Treatment of hypertension slows the progression of chronic kidney disease.

- Angiotensin-converting enzyme (ACE) inhibitors and angiotensin receptor blockers (ARBs) are antihypertensive drugs that have a special advantage for diabetic patients. These antihypertensive drugs have the additional benefit of slowing the progression of kidney disease. For maximum benefit and kidney protection, these drugs are administered at the earliest stage of diabetic kidney disease when microalbuminuria is present.

- To reduce facial or leg swelling, drugs which increase urine volume (diuretics) are given along with restriction of salt and fluid intake.

- Patients with kidney failure due to diabetic kidney disease are prone to hypoglycemia and therefore need modification in drug therapies for diabetes. Short acting insulin is preferred to control diabetes. Avoid long acting oral hypoglycemic agents. Metformin is usually avoided in patients with serum creatinine levels more than 1.5 mg/dl due to the risk of lactic acidosis.

- In diabetic kidney disease with high serum creatinine, all measures of treatment of chronic kidney disease (discussed in Chapter 12) should be followed.

- Evaluate and manage cardiovascular risk factors aggressively (smoking, raised lipids, high blood glucose and high blood pressure).

- Diabetic kidney disease with advanced renal failure requires dialysis or kidney transplant.

Maintain blood pressure less than 130/80 by using ACE inhibitors and ARBs as initial antihypertensive drugs early in the disease.

When should a patient with diabetic kidney disease consult a doctor?

Diabetic patients with microalbuminuria should be referred to a kidney specialist. The patient with diabetic kidney disease should immediately consult a doctor in case of:

- Rapid unexplained weight gain, marked reduction in urine volume, worsening of facial and leg swelling or difficulty in breathing.

- Chest pain, worsening of pre-existing high blood pressure or very slow or fast heart rate.

- Severe weakness, loss of appetite or vomiting or paleness.

- Persistent fever, chills, pain or burning during urination, foul-smelling urine or blood in urine.

- Frequent hypoglycemia (low sugar level) or decreased requirement of insulin or anti-diabetic medications.

- Development of confusion, drowsiness or convulsion.

Meticulous attention to cardiovascular risk factors is an essential part in the management of diabetic kidney disease.

Chapter 16

Polycystic Kidney Disease

Autosomal dominant polycystic kidney disease (ADPKD) is the most common genetic or inherited disease of the kidney, characterized by the growth of numerous cysts in the kidneys. Polycystic kidney disease (PKD) is the fourth leading cause of chronic kidney disease. In PKD, other organs in which cysts can be seen are the liver, brain, intestines, pancreas, ovaries and spleen.

What is the incidence of PKD?

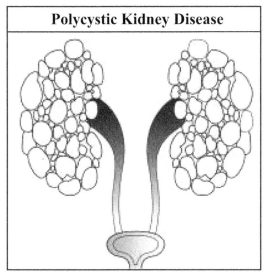

Polycystic Kidney Disease

The incidence of autosomal dominant PKD is the same in all races, occurs equally in males and females and affects about 1 in 1,000 people worldwide. About 5% of all chronic kidney disease patients requiring dialysis or kidney transplantation have PKD.

How is the kidney affected in PKD?

• In autosomal dominant PKD multiple clusters of cysts (fluid-filled sacs) are seen in both kidneys.

• Sizes of cysts in PKD are variable (diameter ranging from a pinhead to as large 10 cm. or more).

Free!!! 200+ Paged Kidney Book in 35+ Languages
Visit: www.KidneyEducation.com

- With time cysts increase in size and slowly compress and damage healthy kidney tissue.

- Such damage leads to hypertension, loss of protein in urine and reduction in kidney function, causing chronic kidney failure.

- In a long period (after years) chronic kidney failure worsens and leads to severe kidney failure (endstage kidney disease), ultimately requiring dialysis or kidney transplantation.

Symptoms of PKD

Many people with autosomal dominant PKD live for several decades without developing symptoms. Most patients with PKD develop symptoms after the age of 30 to 40 years. Common symptoms of PKD are:

- High blood pressure.

- Pain in the back, flank pain on one or both sides and/or a swollen abdomen.

- Feeling a large mass (lump) in abdomen.

- Blood or protein in urine.

- Recurrent urinary tract infections and kidney stones.

- Symptoms of chronic kidney disease due to progressive loss of kidney function.

- Symptoms due to cysts in other parts of the body such as the brain, liver, intestine.

- Complications that can occur in a patient with PKD are brain aneurysm, abdominal wall hernias, infection of liver cysts, diverticulae (pouches) in the colon and heart valve abnormalities. About 10% of PKD patients develop a brain aneurysm. An aneurysm

---

PKD is the most commonly inherited kidney disease and among the leading causes of CKD.

---

is a weakening of the wall of the blood vessel which causes bulging. Brain aneurysms can cause headaches and carry a small risk of rupture that can lead to a stroke or even death.

Does everyone with PKD develop kidney failure?

No. Kidney failure does not occur in all patients with PKD. About 50 % of patients with PKD will have kidney failure by the age of 60, and about 60 % will have kidney failure by the age of 70. The risk factors for progression of CKD in patients with PKD include: larger renal size, younger age at diagnosis, hypertension (particularly before age 35 years), proteinuria (> 300 mgs/day), gross hematuria, male gender, > 3 pregnancies, certain genetic mutations (PKD1 gene mutation), as well as tobacco consumption.

Diagnosis of PKD

Diagnostic tests performed in autosomal dominant PKD are:

- **Ultrasound of the kidneys.** This is the most commonly used diagnostic test for PKD because it is reliable, simple, safe, painless, less costly, and easily identifies cysts in the kidneys.

- **CT or MRI scans:** These tests are more precise but are expensive. These tests may detect smaller cysts that cannot be diagnosed by an ultrasound.

- **Family screening:** PKD is an inherited disease in which each child has a 50:50 chance of developing the disease. So screening of family members of a patient with PKD helps in early diagnosis.

- **Tests to assess effect of PKD on kidney:** Urine test is done to detect the presence of blood or protein in urine. Blood test for creatinine is done to assess and monitor the function of the kidney.

Flank and abdominal pain and blood in urine at the age of 40 is the most common presentation of PKD.

- **Incidental diagnosis:** PKD detected in routine health check up or during ultrasound examination done for another reason.
- **Gene linkage analysis.** This is a very specialized blood test, used to detect which family member carries the PKD gene. This test should be done only if imaging tests do not show anything. As this test is available in very few centers and is very expensive, it is done rarely for diagnostic purposes.

Which family members of PKD patients should be screened for PKD?

Brothers, sisters and children of PKD patients should be screened for PKD. In addition, brothers and sisters of parents from whom the disease is inherited by the patient should be screened.

Will all children of PKD patients carry the risk of developing the same disease?

No. PKD is an inherited disease in which if mother or father has autosomal dominant PKD, the children have a 50% possibility of developing the disorder.

Prevention of PKD

Currently there is no treatment that can prevent formation or slow down the growth of cysts in PKD.

Screening of family members and making an early diagnosis before it sets in has several advantages. Early diagnosis provides an opportunity to treat PKD in a better way. Early diagnosis and treatment of high blood pressure prevents development or aggravation of renal failure in PKD. Lifestyle and dietary modification in PKD patients protects their kidney as well as the heart. The major disadvantage of screening is that

---

PKD is an inherited kidney disease so consider screening of adult family members for PKD.

the person may become very anxious about the disease at a stage when the person neither has the symptoms nor needs any treatment.

Why is it not possible to reduce the incidence of PKD?

PKD is diagnosed usually at the age of 40 years or more. Most people have children before this age and therefore it is not possible to prevent its transmission to the next generation.

Treatment of PKD

PKD is a non-curable disease but why does it need treatment?

- To protect the kidneys and delay progression of chronic kidney disease to end stage kidney disease and thereby prolong survival.

- To control the symptoms and prevent complications.

Important measures in the treatment of PKD:

- The patient is asymptomatic for many years after initial diagnosis and does not require any treatment. Such patients need periodic checkup and monitoring.

- Strict control of high blood pressure will slow down the progression of CKD.

- Control of pain with drugs which will not harm the kidney (such as aspirin or acetaminophen). Recurrent or chronic pain occurs in PKD due to cyst expansion.

- Prompt and adequate treatment of urinary tract infections with appropriate antibiotics.

- Early treatment of kidney stones.

- Plenty of fluid intake, provided the person does not have swelling helps in prevention of urinary tract infections and kidney stones.

Treatment is aimed at delaying progression of CKD and treating kidney infections, stones and abdominal pain.

- Meticulous treatment of chronic kidney disease as discussed in Chapters 10 to 14.
- In a very few patients surgical or radiologic drainage of cysts may be indicated because of pain, bleeding, infection, or obstruction.

When should a patient with PKD consult a doctor?

Patients with PKD should immediately consult a doctor if he or she develops:

- Fever, sudden abdominal pain or red urine.
- Severe or recurrent headaches.
- Accidental injury to enlarged kidneys.
- Chest pain, severe loss of appetite, severe vomiting, severe muscle weakness, confusion, drowsiness, unconsciousness or convulsion.

Asymptomatic person with PKD may not require any treatment for many years initially.

Chapter 17
Living with a Single Kidney

To have a single kidney is a matter of worry. But with a few precautions and healthy lifestyle the person lives a normal life with a single kidney.

What problems will a person with a single kidney likely face in normal life? Why?

Almost all persons are born with two kidneys. But because of extra capacity and a large reserve, even a single (or solitary) kidney is capable of performing normal functions of both kidneys. So a person with a single kidney does not have any problem in routine or sexual activity or strenuous work.

Only one kidney is enough for a normal and active life for a lifetime. In most of the cases of patients born with just one kidney, the diagnosis of single kidney is made accidentally while performing radiological tests for entirely different reasons.

In a few people with a single kidney over long periods (years), possible ill effects include high blood pressure and loss of protein in the urine. Reduction in kidney function is very rare.

What are the causes of a single kidney?

Three common circumstances in which a person has a single kidney are:

1. A person is born with one kidney.
2. One kidney is removed surgically. Important reasons for removal of one kidney are stone disease, cancer, obstruction, pus collection in the kidney or severe traumatic injury.

**A person with a single kidney
lives a normal and active life.**

---

3. One kidney is donated for a kidney transplant.

What are the possibilities of having only one kidney from birth?

Many people are born with a single kidney. The likelihood of having only one kidney from birth is about one out of 750 people. A single kidney is more common in males, and it is usually the left kidney which is missing.

Why are precautions required in people with a single kidney?

People with a single kidney function normally, but can be compared with a two wheeler without a spare wheel.

In the absence of a second kidney, if sudden and severe damage occurs to the solitary functioning kidney, acute kidney failure is bound to occur and all kidney functions will worsen rapidly.

Acute kidney failure can cause many problems and complications and needs prompt attention. Within a short period the severity of problems increases and can cause life threatening complications. Such patients need urgent dialysis. To avoid kidney damage and its consequences, precautions should be taken by all people with a single kidney.

In which circumstances is there a risk of sudden damage to a solitary kidney?

Potential circumstances of sudden and severe damage to a solitary kidney are:

1. Sudden blockage to the flow of urine due to a stone or blood clot in the ureter (the tube that connects the kidney to the urinary bladder). The blockage then causes urine to stop flowing out of the kidney.

Many people are born with a single kidney.

---

2. During abdominal surgery, accidental ligation of the ureter of a solitary kidney will prevent the passage of urine to the bladder and will increase pressure in the kidneys that will further damage the solitary kidney.

3. Injury to a solitary kidney. There is a risk of injury to kidney in heavy contact sports such as boxing, hockey, football, martial arts and wrestling. A single kidney becomes larger and heavier than the normal kidney to cope with the requirements of the body. Such an enlarged kidney is more vulnerable to injury.

What precautions are recommended to protect a single kidney?

People with a single kidney need no treatment. But taking precautions is wise to protect the solitary kidney. Important precautions are:

- Drink a lot of water (about three liters per day).

- Avoid injury to the solitary kidney by avoiding contact sports such as boxing, hockey, football, martial arts and wrestling.

- Prevention and early treatment of stone disease and urinary tract infection.

- Before starting any new treatment or abdominal surgery the doctor should be informed that the patient has a single kidney.

- Control of blood pressure, regular exercise, healthy balanced diet and avoidance of pain killers. Avoid high-protein diets and restrict daily salt (sodium) intake if so advised by the doctor.

- Regular medical check ups. The first and most important advice for a person living with one kidney is to have regular medical checkups.

Persons with a single kidney should not worry but need proper precautions and regular medical checkups.

Monitor kidney function by checking blood pressure and testing urine and blood once a year. Regular medical checkups will help detect any early signs of kidney problems or developing kidney failure. Early detection of kidney problems provides opportunity for timely treatment and care.

When should a patient with a single kidney consult a doctor?

Patients with a single kidney should immediately consult a doctor if there is:

- A sudden decrease or total absence of urine output.
- Accidental injury to an enlarged solitary kidney.
- A need to take medicine for pain.
- A need to use X-ray dyes for diagnostic tests.
- Fever, burning urination or red urine.

Sudden decrease and total absence of urine output occurs usually due to stone-induced obstruction.

The urinary system is normally composed of two kidneys, two ureters, a single urinary bladder and a single urethra. Urinary tract infection (UTI) is a bacterial infection that affects any part of the urinary tract. UTI is the second most common type of infection in the body.

What are the symptoms of a urinary tract infection?

The symptoms of urinary tract infections may vary with severity of infection, age and location of infection in the tract.

Most Common Symptoms of urinary tract infection

- Burning or pain during urination.
- Frequency of urination and persistent urge to urinate.
- Fever and malaise.
- Foul odor and cloudy urine.

Symptoms due to infection of the urinary bladder (Cystitis)

- Lower abdomen discomfort.
- Frequent, painful urination with small amounts of urine.
- Usually low-grade fever without flank pain.
- Blood in urine.

Symptoms due to infection of upper urinary tract (Pyelonephritis)

- Upper back and flank pain.

> **Burning and frequent urination are common signs of urinary tract infection.**

- High grade fever with chills.
- Nausea, vomiting, weakness, fatigue and general ill-feeling.
- Mental changes or confusion in elderly people.

This is the most serious symptom of urinary tract infection as it implies systemic involvement. Inadequate and delayed treatment can be life threatening.

What are the causes of recurrent urinary tract infection?

Important causes of frequent or recurrent urinary tract infections are:

1. **Urinary tract obstruction:** Various underlying causes which can lead to obstruction of urinary tract.

2. **Female gender:** Because of shorter urethra, women are more susceptible than men to UTI.

3. **Intercourse:** Women who are sexually active tend to have more urinary tract infections than women who aren't sexually active.

4. **Urinary stones:** Kidney, ureter or bladder stone can block the flow of urine and increases risk for UTI.

5. **Urinary catheterization:** People with indwelling catheters have an increased risk of UTI.

6. **Congenital urinary tract anomalies:** Children with congenital urinary tract anomalies such as vesicoureteral reflux (condition in which urine moves backward from the bladder up the ureters) and posterior urethral valve have an increased risk of UTI.

7. **Benign prostatic hyperplasia:** Men over 60 years are prone to UTI because of an enlarged prostate (benign prostatic hyperplasia - BPH).

8. **Suppressed immune systems:** Patients with diabetes, HIV or cancer are at higher risk for UTI.

**Obstruction of urinary tract is
an important cause of recurrent UTI.**

---

9. Other causes: Narrowing of the urethra or ureters, tuberculosis of the genito-urinary tract, neurogenic bladder or bladder diverticulum.

Can recurrent urinary tract infection cause damage to the kidney?

Recurrent lower urinary tract infection usually does not cause damage to kidneys in adults.

UTI in adults can cause damage to the kidneys if predisposing factors such as stone, blockage or narrowing of flow of urine and tuberculosis of the genito-urinary tract are not corrected.

However, in young children, delayed or improper treatment of recurrent urinary tract infection can cause irreversible damage to the growing kidney especially in those with vesicoureteral reflux. This damage may lead to reduction of kidney function and high blood pressure later in life. So the problem of urinary tract infection is more serious in children compared to adults.

Diagnosis of Urinary Tract Infection

Investigations are performed to establish diagnosis and severity of urinary tract infection. In a person with complicated or recurrent urinary tract infection different tests are performed to establish the presence of predisposing or risk factors.

Basic Investigations for Urine Tract Infection

1. Urine test

Most important screening test for UTI is routine urinalysis. Early morning urine sample is preferable for this test. In microscopic examination of urine, presence of significant white blood cells is suggestive of UTI.

> **UTI does not usually cause permanent damage to the kidneys in adults in the absence of blockage of urine flow.**

Presence of white blood cells in urine suggests inflammation of the urinary tract but its absence does not exclude UTI.

Special urine dipstick (leukocyte esterase and nitrite) tests are useful screening tests for UTI that can be done at the office or home. A positive urine dipstick test suggests UTI and such patients need further evaluation. The intensity of color change is proportional to the number of bacteria in the urine.

2. Urine culture and sensitivity test

The gold standard for the diagnosis of UTI is a urine culture test and it should be done before starting antibiotic therapy. A urine culture is recommended in complicated or resistant UTI and, in a few cases, for the confirmation of the clinical diagnosis of urinary tract infection.

Urine culture test results are available after 48-72 hours. The significant time delay between collection of sample and availability of the report is a major drawback of this test. Urine culture identifies the specific bacteria causing infection based on the nature of growth of the organism and the number of colony forming units that grow in the Petri dish in the laboratory. The urine culture result also includes the type of antibiotics that the organism grown may be sensitive or resistant to. This guides the doctor in the appropriate choice of antibiotic.

To avoid potential contamination of the urine sample, the patient is asked first to clean the genital area and to collect midstream urine in a sterile container. Other methods used for sample collection for urine culture are supra-pubic aspiration, catheter-specimen urine and bag specimen urine.

> **Urine culture and sensitivity is a valuable test for the diagnosis and treatment of UTI.**

3. Blood tests

Blood tests usually performed in a patient with UTI include a complete blood count (CBC), blood urea, serum creatinine, blood sugar and C reactive protein.

Investigations to Identify Predisposing or Risk Factors

If the infection does not respond to treatment or if there is repetition of infections, further investigations, as mentioned below, are required to detect underlying predisposing or risk factors:

1. Ultrasound and X-rays of the abdomen.

2. CT scan or MRI of the abdomen.

3. Voiding cystourethrogram - VCUG (Micturating cystourethrogram – MCU).

4. Intravenous urography (IVU).

5. Microscopic examination of urine for tuberculosis.

6. Cystoscopy - a procedure in which a urologist (kidney surgeon) looks inside the bladder using a special instrument called a cystoscope.

7. Examination by a gynecologist.

8. Urodynamics.

9. Blood Cultures.

Prevention of Urinary Tract Infection

1. Drink plenty (3-4 liters) of fluids daily. Fluids dilute urine and help in flushing bacteria out of the bladder and urinary tract.

2. Urinate every two to three hours. Do not postpone going to the

---

For successful treatment of UTI, it is essential to identify underlying predisposing factors.

bathroom. Holding urine in the bladder for a long period provides opportunity for bacteria to grow.

3. Consume food containing vitamin C, ascorbic acid or cranberry juice to make urine acidic eventually reducing bacterial growth.

4. Avoid constipation or treat it promptly.

5. Women and girls should wipe from front to back (not back to front) after using the toilet. This habit prevents bacteria in the anal region from spreading to the vagina and urethra.

6. Clean genital and anal areas before and after intercourse. Urinate before and after intercourse and drink a full glass of water soon after intercourse.

7. Women should wear only cotton undergarments, which allow air circulation. Avoid tight-fitting pants and nylon underwear.

8. Recurrent urinary tract infection in women after sexual activity can be effectively prevented by taking a single dose of an appropriate antibiotic after sexual contact.

Treatment of Urinary Tract Infection

General measures

Drink plenty of water. A person who is very ill, dehydrated or unable to take adequate oral fluids due to vomiting, will need hospitalization and administration of IV fluids.

Take medications to reduce fever and pain. Use of heating pad reduces pain. Avoid coffee, alcohol, smoking and spicy foods, all of which irritate the bladder. Follow all preventive measures of urinary tract infection.

It is essential to drink plenty of water to prevent and treat urinary tract infection.

Treatment of lower urinary tract infection (cystitis, mild infections)

In a healthy young female, short term antibiotics for three days is usually enough. Some drugs need to be given for seven days to complete a course. Occasionally, a single dose of an antibiotic such as Fosfomycin can be used. Except for a previously healthy adult male who develops a cystitis for the first time, adult males with UTI require 7 to 14 days of antibiotics because of underlying structural abnormalities of the urinary tract that make them prone to infection. Commonly used oral antibiotics are nitrofurantoin, trimethoprim, cephalosporins, or fluoroquinolones. The choice of antibiotic is best determined by the sensitivity and resistance patterns of commonly used drugs in your locality.

Treatment of severe kidney infection (Pyelonephritis)

Patients with moderate-to-severe acute kidney infection, those with severe symptoms or sick patients need hospitalization. Urine and blood cultures are obtained before initiating therapy to identify causative bacteria and proper selection of antibiotics. Patients are treated with intravenous fluids and antibiotics for several days, followed by 10-14 days of oral antibiotics. If response to IV antibiotics is poor (marked by persistent symptoms and fever, worsening kidney function) imaging is indicated. Follow up urine tests are necessary to assess response to therapy.

Treatment of recurrent urinary tract infection

In patients with recurrent UTI, proper identification of the underlying cause is essential. According to the underlying cause, specific medical or surgical treatment is planned. These patients need follow-up, strict adherence to preventive measures and long term preventive antibiotic therapy.

Treatment of severe kidney infections (pyelonephritis) requires hospitalization and intravenous antibiotics.

When should a patient with UTI consult a doctor?

All children with UTI should be evaluated by a doctor. Adult patients with UTI should immediately consult a doctor when there is:

- Decrease in urine volume or total absence of urine output.
- Persistent high fever, chills, back pain and cloudy urine or blood in the urine.
- No response to antibiotics after 2 to 3 days of treatment.
- Severe vomiting, severe weakness or fall of blood pressure.
- A single kidney.
- Previous history of stones.

Persistent high fever, chills, back pain, cloudy urine, burning sensation need urgent attention.

Stone disease is a very common urological disease. Kidney stones can cause the most unbearable pain, but sometimes kidney stones can exist silently without any symptom. Stone disease can cause urinary tract infection and can damage the kidney if not treated adequately. Once a stone occurs, its recurrence is common. So understanding, prevention and care of stone disease is essential.

What is a kidney stone?

A kidney stone is a hard crystal mass formed within the kidney or urinary tract. Increased concentration of crystals or small particles of calcium, oxalate, urate, or phosphate in urine is responsible for stone formation. Millions of crystals of these substances in urine aggregate, gradually increase in size, and after a long period of time, form a stone.

Normally, urine contains substances that prevent or inhibit the aggregation of crystals. Reduced levels of stone inhibitor substances contribute to the formation of kidney stones. Urolithiasis is the medical term used to describe urinary stones. It is to be noted that the composition of gall stones (found in the gall bladder) and kidney stones is different.

What are the size, shape and location of urinary stones?

Kidney stones vary in size and shape. They can be smaller than a grain of sand or can be as large as a tennis ball. The shape of the stone may be round or oval with a smooth surface, or they can be irregular or jagged with a rough surface. Stones with a smooth surface cause less pain and their chances of natural removal are high. On the other hand, kidney stones that have an irregular rough surface can cause more pain

---

Stones in the urinary tract are an important cause of unbearable abdominal pain.

---

and are less likely to come out on their own. Stones can occur anywhere in the urinary system but occur more frequently in the kidney and then descend into the ureter, sometimes lodging in the narrow areas of the ureter.

What are the types of kidney stones?

There are four main types of kidney stones:

1. Calcium Stones: This is the most common type of kidney stone, which occurs in about 70 - 80% of cases. Calcium stones are usually composed of calcium oxalate and less commonly, of calcium phosphate. Calcium oxalate stones are relatively hard and difficult to dissolve with medical management. Calcium phosphate stones are found in alkaline urine.

2. Struvite Stones: Struvite (Magnesium ammonium phosphate) stones are less common (about 10 - 15%) and result from infections in the kidney. A struvite stone is more common in women and grows only in alkaline urine.

3. Uric Acid Stones: Uric acid stones are not very common (about 5 - 10%) and are more likely to form when there is too much uric acid in the urine and urine is persistently acidic. Uric acid stones can form in people with gout, who eat a high animal protein diet, are dehydrated or have undergone chemotherapy. Uric acid stones are radiolucent, so are not detected by an X-ray of the abdomen.

4. Cystine Stones: Cystine stones are rare and occur in an inherited condition called cystinuria. Cystinuria is characterized by high levels of cystine in the urine.

> **Urinary stone occurs most frequently in the kidney and ureter.**

What is a staghorn stone?

A staghorn calculus is a very large stone, usually struvite, occupying a large part of the kidney and resembling the horns of a stag (deer), thus it is called staghorn. A staghorn stone causes minimal or even no pain, diagnosis is missed in most of the cases and end result is damage to kidney.

Which factors contribute to the formation of urinary stone?

Everyone is susceptible to stone formation. Several factors that increase the risk of developing kidney stones are:

• Reduced fluid - especially decreased water intake and dehydration.

• Family history of kidney stones.

• Diet: consuming a diet high in animal protein, sodium and oxalate, but low in fiber and potassium rich citrus fruits.

• 75 % of kidney stones and 95% of bladder stones occur in men. Men between the age of 20 to 70 years and those who are obese are most vulnerable.

• A person who is bed-ridden or immobile for a long period.

• A person living in a hot humid atmosphere.

• Recurrent urinary tract infections and blockage to the flow of urine.

• Metabolic diseases: hyperparathyroidism, cystinuria, gout etc.

• Use of certain medications such as diuretics and antacids.

What are the symptoms of a urinary stone?

The symptoms of urinary stone may vary with size, shape, and location of the urinary stone. Common symptoms of urinary stone are:

Reduced water intake and family history of kidney stones are two most important risk factors for stone formation.

- Abdominal pain.

- No symptoms. Accidental detection of urinary stone on routine health checkups or during the workup for unrelated conditions. Stones that do not cause any symptoms and are detected accidentally on radiological examinations are known as "silent stones."

- Frequency of urination and persistent urge to urinate is found in patients with a urinary bladder stone.

- Nausea or vomiting.

- Passage of blood in urine (hematuria).

- Pain and/or burning while passing urine.

- If the bladder stone gets stuck at the entrance to the urethra, the flow of urine suddenly stops during urination.

- Passage of stones in urine.

- In a few cases urinary stones can cause complications such as recurrent urinary tract infection and obstruction of the urinary tract, causing temporary or permanent damage to the kidney.

Characteristics of abdominal pain due to urinary stone

- The severity and the location of the pain can vary from person to person depending upon the type, the size and the position of the stone within the urinary tract. Remember, the size of the stone does not correlate with the severity of pain. Smaller-sized rough stones usually cause more severe pain than bigger-sized smooth stones.

- Stone pain can vary from a vague flank pain to the sudden onset of severe unbearable pain. Pain is aggravated by change of posture and vehicular jerks. The pain may last for minutes to hours followed by relief. Waxing and waning of pain is characteristic of a stone passing down the ureter.

Abdominal pain and blood in urine strongly indicate the presence of urinary stones.

- The abdominal pain occurs on the side where the stone is lodged. Classical pain of kidney and ureteric stone is the pain from loin to groin and is usually accompanied by nausea and vomiting.

- A bladder stone may also cause lower abdominal pain and pain during urination, which is often felt at the tip of the penis in males.

- Many people who experience sudden severe abdominal pain from stone in the urinary tract rush to seek immediate medical attention.

Can kidney stones damage the kidney?

Yes. Stones in the kidney or ureter can block or obstruct the flow of urine within the urinary tract. Such obstruction can cause dilatation of the urinary pelvis and calyces in the kidney. Persistent severe dilatation due to blockage can cause kidney damage in the long term in a few patients.

Diagnosis of urinary stones

Investigations are performed not only to establish diagnosis of urinary stones and to detect complications but also to identify factors which promote stone formation.

Radiological investigations

KUB Ultrasound: The KUB ultrasound is an easily available, less expensive and simple test that is used most commonly for the diagnosis of urinary stones and to detect the presence of obstruction.

KUB X-ray : Size, shape and position of the urinary stones can be seen on the X-ray of the kidney-ureter-bladder (KUB). A KUB X-ray is the most useful method to monitor presence and size of stone before and after treatment of calcium containing stones.It cannot be used to identify radiolucent stones such as those containing uric acid.

Beware of "Silent Stones" which cause no pain, but are most likely to cause kidney damage.

CT scan: CT scan of the urinary system is an extremely accurate and the most preferred diagnostic method to identify stones of all sizes and to determine the presence of obstruction.

Intravenous urography (IVU): Less frequently used, IVU is very reliable in detecting stones and obstruction. The major benefit of IVU is that it provides information about the function of the kidney. Structure of the kidney and details about ureteric dilatation is better judged by this test. It is not useful and should not be used when the serum creatinine is elevated.

Laboratory investigations

Urine tests: Urine tests to detect infection and to measure pH of the urine; 24 hour urine collection to measure total daily urine volume, calcium, phosphorous, uric acid, magnesium, oxalate, citrate, sodium and creatinine.

Blood tests: Basic tests such as complete blood count, serum creatinine, electrolytes and blood sugar; and special tests to identify certain chemicals which promote stone formation such as calcium, phosphorus, uric acid and level of parathyroid hormone.

Stone analysis: Stones that pass out or are removed by different treatment modalities should be collected for analysis. Chemical analysis of stones can establish their composition, which helps in treatment planning.

Prevention of urinary stones

"Once a kidney stone former, always a stone former." Urinary stones recur in about 50 to 70% of persons. On the other hand, with proper precautions and treatment the recurrence rate can be reduced to 10% or less. Thus, all patients who suffer from kidney stones should follow preventive measures.

> **For diagnosis of stones in the urinary tract, CT scan, sonography and X ray are the most important investigations.**

General measures

Diet is an important factor that can promote or inhibit formation of urinary stones. General measures useful to all patients with urinary stones are:

1. Drink lots of fluid

- A simple and most important measure to prevent formation of stone is to drink plenty of water, drink plenty of water and drink plenty of water. Drink 12 - 14 glasses (more than 3 liters) of water per day. To ensure adequate water intake throughout the day, carry a water bottle with you.

- Which water to drink is a dilemma for many patients. But remember, to prevent formation of stone the quantity of water is more important than the quality of water.

- For stone prevention, formation of a sufficient volume of urine per day is more important than the volume of fluid taken. To ensure that you are drinking enough water, measure the total volume of urine per day. It should be more than 2 - 2.5 liters per day.

- Urine color or concentration may suggest how much water you are drinking. If you drink enough water throughout the day, the urine will be diluted, clear and almost watery. Diluted urine suggests a low concentration of minerals, which prevents stone formation. Yellow, dark, concentrated urine suggests inadequate water intake.

- To prevent stone formation make it a habit to drink two glasses of water after each meal. It is particularly important to drink two glasses of water before going to bed and an additional glass at each night time awakening. If you need to wake up several times during the night to urinate, you have probably drunk enough fluids during the

---

Plenty of fluid intake is the simplest and most essential measure for prevention and treatment of urinary stone.

---

day and night.

- Higher fluid intake is recommended in physically active people on hot days, because a significant amount of water is lost through perspiration.

- Intake of fluids such as coconut water, barley or rice water, citrate-rich fluids such as lemonade and pineapple juice, helps in increasing total fluid intake and prevention of stone.

Which fluids are preferred to prevent urinary stone?

Intake of fluids such as coconut water, barley or rice water and citrate-rich fluids such as lemonade, tomato juice or pineapple fruit juices helps in the prevention of stone. But remember that at least 50% of the total fluid intake should be water.

Which fluids should be avoided by a person with urinary stone?

Avoid grapefruit, cranberry and apple juice; strong tea, coffee, chocolate and sugar sweetened soft drinks such as colas; and all alcoholic beverages, including beer. These beverages have been associated with an increased risk of stone formation.

2. Salt restriction

Avoid excessive salt intake in diet. Avoid pickles, chips and salty snacks. Excessive quantities of salt or sodium in the diet can increase the excretion of calcium into the urine and thereby increase the risk of formation of calcium stones. Sodium intake should be restricted to less than 100 mEq or 6 grams table salt per day to prevent stone formation.

3. Decrease intake of animal protein

Avoid non-vegetarian food such as mutton, chicken, fish and egg. These

---

Clean, transparent, water- like urine denotes adequate fluid intake.

---

animal foods contain high uric acid/purines and can increase the risk of uric acid and calcium stones.

4. Balanced diet

Eat a balanced diet with more vegetables and fruits that reduces acid load and tend to make urine less acidic. Eat fruits such as banana, pineapple, blueberries, cherries, and oranges. Eat vegetables such as carrots, bitter gourd (karela-ampalaya), squash and bell peppers. Eat high-fiber containing foods such as barley, beans, oats, and psyllium seed. Avoid or restrict refined foods such as white bread, pastas, and sugar. Kidney stones are associated with high sugar intake.

5. Other advice

Restrict intake of vitamin C to less than 1000 mg per day. Avoid large meals late at night. Obesity is an independent risk factor for stone formation.

Special measures

1. To prevent calcium stone

- Diet: It is a wrong concept that calcium should be avoided by patients suffering from kidney stones. Eat a healthy diet with calcium, including dairy products, to prevent stone formation. Dietary calcium binds with oxalate in the gut which limits intestinal oxalate absorption and subsequently reduces stone formation. On the other hand, when dietary calcium is reduced, unbound oxalate in the gut can be easily absorbed from the intestines to promote formation of oxalate stones.

- Avoid calcium supplements as well as a diet that is low in calcium, because both increase the risk of stone development. Dietary sources

---

Restriction of salt intake in diet is very important for the prevention of calcium stones.

---

of calcium such as dairy products are preferred over oral calcium supplements for patients at risk for the development of kidney stones. If oral calcium supplements are necessary, they should be taken with meals to reduce the risk.

- Medication: Thiazide diuretics are helpful in the prevention of calcium stones because they limit the excretion of calcium in the urine.

2. To prevent oxalate stone

People with calcium oxalate stones should limit foods high in oxalate. Foods rich in oxalate include:

- Vegetables: spinach, rhubarb, okra, (lady finger), beets and sweet potatoes.
- Fruits and dry fruits: strawberries, raspberries, chiku, amla, custard apples, grapes, cashew nuts, peanuts, almonds and dried figs.
- Other foods: green pepper, fruit cake, marmalade, dark chocolate, peanut butter, soybean foods and cocoa.
- Drinks: grapefruit juice, dark colas, and strong or black tea.

3. To prevent uric acid stone

- Avoid all alcoholic beverages.
- Avoid foods high in animal protein such as organ meat (e.g. as brain, liver, kidney), fish especially those without scales (e.g. anchovies, sardines, herring, trout salmon), pork, chicken, beef and egg.
- Restrict pulses, legumes like beans or lentils; vegetables like mushrooms, spinach, asparagus and cauliflower.
- Restrict fatty foods such as salad dressings, ice cream, and fried foods.

Beware. Restriction of calcium in the diet will promote stone formation!

- Medication: Allopurinol to inhibit uric acid synthesis and decrease urinary uric acid excretion. Potassium citrate to maintain urine alkaline, as uric acid precipitates and forms stones in acidic urine.

- Other measures: weight reduction. Obese patients are not able to alkalinize urine and this increases the risk for the formation of uric acid stones.

Treatment of urinary stones

Factors determining the treatment of urinary stones depend on the degree of symptoms; size, position and cause of stone; and presence or absence of urinary infection and obstruction. Two major treatment options are:

A. Conservative treatment

B. Surgical treatment

A. Conservative Treatment

Most kidney stones are small (less than 5 mm in diameter) enough to pass on their own within 3 to 6 weeks of the onset of symptoms. The aim of conservative treatment is to relieve symptoms and to help stone removal without surgical operation.

Immediate treatment of kidney stones

To treat unbearable pain a patient may require intramuscular or intravenous administration of non-steroidal inflammatory drugs (NSAIDs) or opioids. For less severe pain, oral medications are often effective.

Plenty of fluid intake

In patients with severe pain, fluid intake should be moderate and not excessive because it may aggravate pain. But in pain free periods,

---

Plenty of fluid intake will flush out a large number of small stones in urine.

---

138. *Save Your Kidneys*

drink plenty of fluids, taking as much as 2 to 3 liters of water in a day. Remember though that beer is NOT a therapeutic agent for a patient with kidney stones.

Patients with severe colic and associated nausea, vomiting and fever may require intravenous saline infusion to correct fluid deficit. Patient must save the passed out stone for testing. A simple way to collect stones that have passed out is to urinate through a strainer (sieve).

Other measures

Maintaining proper urine pH is essential especially for patients with uric acid stone. Drugs like calcium channel blockers and alpha-blockers inhibit spasms of the ureter and dilate the ureters sufficiently to allow the passage of the ureteral stone. This is particularly helpful when the stone is located in the ureter close to the urinary bladder. Treat associated problems such as nausea, vomiting and urinary tract infection. Follow all general and special preventive measures (dietary advice, medication etc) discussed.

B. Surgical Treatment

Different surgical treatments are available for kidney stones that cannot be treated with conservative measures. Most frequently used surgical methods are extra-corporeal shock wave lithotripsy (ESWL), percutaneous nephrolithotripsy (PCNL), ureteroscopy and in rare cases open surgery. These techniques are complimentary to each other. These procedures are performed by the urologist who decides which method is the best for a particular patient.

Which patient, with urinary stone, needs surgical treatment?

Most patients with small stones can be effectively treated conservatively. But surgery may be needed to remove kidney stones when the stones:

Stone recurs in more than 50% cases. Instructions for prevention are emphatically advised.

Free!!! 200+ Paged Kidney Book in 35+ Languages
Visit: www.KidneyEducation.com

- Cause recurrent or severe pain and do not pass out after a reasonable period of time.

- Are too large to pass on their own. Stones > 6 mm may need surgical intervention.

- Cause significant obstruction, blocking the flow of urine and damaging the kidney.

- Cause recurrent urinary tract infection or bleeding.

Prompt surgery may be required in patients with kidney failure due to stone obstructing the only functioning kidney or both the kidneys simultaneously.

1. ESWL - Extra-Corporeal Shockwave Lithotripsy

ESWL or extra-corporeal shock wave lithotripsy is the latest, effective and most frequently used treatment for kidney stones. Lithotripsy is ideal for kidney stones less than 1.5 cm in size or upper ureteric stones.

In lithotripsy highly concentrated shock waves or ultrasonic waves produced by a lithotriptor machine break up the stones. The stones break down into small particles and are easily passed out through the urinary tract in the urine. After lithotripsy, the patient is advised to drink fluids liberally to flush out stone fragments. When blockage of the ureter is anticipated after lithotripsy of a big stone, a "stent" (special soft plastic tube) is placed in the ureter to avoid blockage.

Lithotripsy is generally safe. Probable complications of lithotripsy are blood in urine, urinary tract infection, incomplete stone removal (may require more sessions), incomplete stone fragmentation (which can lead to urinary tract obstruction), damage to kidney and an elevation in blood pressure.

> **Lithotripsy is an effective and most frequently used non-operative treatment for kidney stones.**

Advantages of lithotripsy are that it is a safe method that does not require hospitalization, anesthesia and incision or cut. Pain is minimum in this method and it is suitable for patients of all age groups.

Lithotripsy is less effective for large stones and in obese patients. Lithotripsy is not advisable during pregnancy and in patients with severe infection, uncontrolled hypertension, distal obstruction in the urinary tract and bleeding disorders.

After lithotripsy, regular follow up, periodical checkup and strict adherence to preventive measures against recurrence of stone disease, is mandatory.

2. Percutaneous Nephrolithotomy (PCNL)

Percutaneous nephrolithotomy, or PCNL, is an effective method for removing medium-sized or large (bigger than 1.5 cm) kidney or ureteral stones. PCNL is the most frequently used option when other treatment modalities such as ureteroscopy or lithotripsy have failed.

In this procedure, under general anesthesia, the urologist makes a tiny incision in the back and creates a small tract from the skin to the kidney under image intensifier or sonographic control. For the insertion of instruments the tract is dilated. Using an instrument called a nephroscope, the urologist locates and removes the stone (nephrolithotomy). When the stone is big it is broken up using high frequency sound waves and then the stone fragments are removed (nephrolithotripsy).

By and large PCNL is safe, but there are some risks and complications that can arise as with any surgical treatment. Probable complications of PCNL are bleeding, infection, injury to other abdominal organs such as the colon, urinary leak and hydrothorax.

PCNL is the most effective method for removal of medium or large-sized kidney stones.

The main advantage of PCNL is that only a small incision (about one centimeter) is required. For all types of stones, PCNL is the most effective modality to make the patient totally stone-free in a single sitting. With PCNL hospital stay is shorter and recovery and healing is faster.

3. Ureteroscopy (URS)

Ureteroscopy is a highly successful modality for treating stones located in the mid and lower ureter. Under anaesthesia, a thin lighted flexible tube (ureteroscope) equipped with a camera is inserted via the urethra into the bladder and up the ureter.

The stone is seen through the ureteroscope and, depending on the size of the stone and the diameter of the ureter, the stone may be fragmented and/or removed. If the ureteric stone is small, it is grasped by the grasper and removed. If a stone is too large to remove in one piece, it can be broken into tiny fragments using pneumatic lithotripsy. These tiny stone pieces pass out on their own in urine. Patients normally go home the same day and can resume normal activity in two to three days.

The advantages of URS are that even hard stones can be broken by this method, and that it does not require incisions. It is safe for pregnant women, obese persons, as well as those with bleeding disorders.

URS is generally safe, but, as with any procedure, risks exist. Possible complications of URS are blood in the urine, urinary tract infection, perforation of the ureter, and formation of scar tissue that narrows the diameter of the ureter (ureteral stricture).

4. Open Surgery

Open surgery is the most invasive and painful treatment modality for stone disease requiring five to seven days of hospitalization.

> **Mid and lower ureteric stones can be successfully removed by ureteroscopy without surgery.**

With the availability of new technologies, the need for open surgery has been reduced drastically. At present, open surgery is used only in extremely rare situations for very complicated cases with very large stone burden.

Major benefit of open surgery is complete removal of multiple, very big or staghorn stones in a single sitting. Open surgery is an efficient and cost-effective treatment modality especially for developing countries where resources are limited.

When should a patient with kidney stone consult a doctor?

A patient with kidney stone should immediately consult a doctor in case of:

- Severe pain in the abdomen not relieved with medication.
- Severe nausea or vomiting which prevents intake of fluid and medication.
- Fever, chills and burning urination with pain in abdomen.
- Blood in urine.
- No urine output.

Reserve open surgery for very few patients with very large kidney stones or when other modalities have failed.

Chapter 20

Benign Prostatic Hyperplasia (BPH)

The prostate gland is present only in males. Enlargement of the prostate gland causes problems in urination in elderly male. (usually over the age of 60 years). With increase in life expectancy, the incidence of benign prostatic hyperplasia (also called BPH) has also increased.

What is the prostate gland? What is its function?

The prostate gland is a small organ about the size of a walnut and is part of the male reproductive system.

The prostate gland is situated just underneath the bladder and in front of the rectum. It surrounds the initial portion of the urethra (the tube that carries urine from the bladder). In other words, the initial portion of the urethra (about 3 cm. long) runs through the prostate.

The prostate is a male reproductive organ. It secretes fluid that nourishes and carries sperm into the urethra during ejaculation.

What is benign prostatic hyperplasia (BPH)?

"Benign prostatic" means the prostatic problem is not caused by cancer and **"hyperplasia"** means enlargement.

Benign prostatic hyperplasia or benign prostatic hypertrophy (BPH) is a non-cancerous prostatic enlargement that occurs in almost all men as they get older. As men age, the prostate gland slowly grows bigger (or enlarges). An enlarged prostate compresses the urethra, blocks the urine stream and causes problems in urination. Because of narrowing of the urethra, flow of urine becomes slower and less forceful.

Benign Prostatic Hyperplasia is a disease of elderly males.

Symptoms of BPH

The symptoms of BPH usually begin after age 50. More than half of men in their 60s and up to 90% of men in their 70s and 80s have symptoms of BPH. Most symptoms of BPH start gradually and worsen over the years. The most common symptoms of BPH are:

- Frequent urination, especially at night. This is usually a very early symptom.
- Slow or weak stream of urine.
- Difficulty or straining in starting the urine flow, even when the bladder feels full.
- Urge to urinate immediately is the most bothersome symptom.
- Straining to urinate.
- Interrupted urine flow.
- Leaking or dribbling at the end of urination. Drops of urine are expelled even after urination causing wetting of underclothes.
- Incomplete emptying of bladder.

Complications of BPH

Severe BPH can cause serious problems over a time in a few patients, if left untreated. Common complications of BPH are:

- **Acute urinary retention:** untreated severe BPH over time can cause sudden, complete and often painful blockage of urine flow. Such patients require insertion of a tube called a catheter to drain urine from the bladder.
- **Chronic urinary retention:** partial blockage of urine flow for a prolonged period can cause chronic urinary retention. Chronic urinary retention is painless and is characterized by an increased residual

---

BPH causes weak stream of urine and frequent urination, especially at night.

---

urine volume. The amount of urine which remains in bladder after normal urination is called residual urine. Its usual presentation is incomplete bladder emptying or frequent voiding of small amount of urine (overflow of urine).

- **Damage to bladder and kidney:** chronic urinary retention causes stretching of the muscular wall of the bladder. In the long term the bladder becomes weak and no longer contracts properly.

  Large residual urine volume leads to increased pressure in the bladder. High bladder pressure may lead to a back pressure of urine through the ureters and into the kidneys. Resultant fullness of the ureters and the kidneys eventually may lead to kidney failure.

- **Urinary tract infection and bladder stones:** inability to completely empty the bladder increases the risk of urinary tract infection and formation of bladder stones.

- Remember, BPH does not increase the risk for prostate cancer.

Diagnosis of BPH

When history and symptoms suggest BPH, the following tests are performed to confirm or rule out the presence of an enlarged prostate.

- **Digital rectal examination (DRE)**

In this examination, a lubricated, gloved finger is gently inserted into the patient's rectum to feel the surface of the prostate gland through the rectal wall. This examination gives the doctor an idea of the size and condition of the prostate gland.

In BPH, on DRE, the prostate is enlarged, smooth, and firm in consistency. Hard, nodular and irregular feel of the prostate on DRE suggests cancer or calcification of prostate gland.

Digital rectal examination and sonography are two most important tests for the diagnosis of BPH.

- **Ultrasound and post-void residual volume test**

An ultrasound can estimate the size of the prostate and detect other problems such as malignancy, dilatation of the ureter and the presence of a kidney abscess.

Ultrasound imaging is also used to determine the quantity of urine left in the bladder after urination. Post-void residual urine volume less than 50 ml indicates adequate bladder emptying. Post-void residual urine volume of 100 to 200 ml or higher is considered to be significant and further evaluation is needed.

- **Prostate symptom score or index**

The International Prostate Symptom Score (IPSS) or AUA (American Urological Association) symptom index helps in the diagnosis of BPH. In this diagnostic modality, patients are asked about the presence or absence of common symptoms of benign prostatic hyperplasia. The answers are then scored and, on the basis of the calculated prostate symptoms score, the severity of the urinary problem is judged.

- **Laboratory tests**

Laboratory tests do not help diagnosing of BPH. But they help in the diagnosis of associated complications and excluding problems with similar presentation. Urine is tested for infection and blood is tested for kidney function.

Prostate Specific Antigen (PSA) is a screening blood test for cancer of the prostate.

- **Other investigations**

Different investigations performed to diagnose or exclude the diagnosis of BPH are uroflowmetry, urodynamic studies, cystoscopy, prostate

---

Blood PSA test is an important screening test for the diagnosis of cancer of the prostate.

---

biopsy, intravenous pyelogram or CT urogram and retrograde pyelography.

Can a person with symptoms of BPH have prostate cancer? How is prostate cancer diagnosed?

Yes. Many symptoms of prostate cancer and BPH are similar, so on the basis of clinical symptoms it is not possible to differentiate between the two conditions. But remember, BPH is not related to prostate cancer. Three most important tests which can establish the diagnosis of prostate cancer are digital rectal examination (DRE), blood test for prostate-specific antigen (PSA) and prostate biopsy.

Treatment of BPH

Factors determining treatment options of BPH are severity of symptoms, the extent to which daily life is affected due to symptoms, and the presence of associated medical conditions. Goals of treatment of BPH are to reduce symptoms, improve quality of life, reduce post void residual urine volume and prevent complications of BPH.

Three different treatment options of BPH are:

A. Watchful waiting and lifestyle changes (no treatment)

B. Medical Treatment

C. Surgical Treatment

A. Watchful waiting and lifestyle changes (no treatment)

"Wait and watch" without any treatment is the preferred approach for men with mild symptoms or symptoms that don't bother them. But watchful waiting does not mean to simply wait and do nothing to reduce symptoms of BPH. During watchful waiting, the person should make

---

Many symptoms of prostate cancer and BPH are similar. Thorough investigation is required for accurate diagnosis.

---

changes in life style to reduce symptoms of BPH and also have regular yearly checkups to see if the symptoms are improving or getting worse.

- Make simple changes in the habits of urination and in consumption of liquids.

- Empty bladder regularly. Do not hold back urine for long. Urinate as soon as the urge arises.

- Double void. This means urine is passed twice in succession. First empty the bladder normally in a relaxed way, wait for a few moments, and try to void again. Do not strain or push to empty.

- Avoid drinking alcohol and caffeine containing beverages in the evening. Both can affect the muscle tone of the bladder, and both stimulate the kidneys to produce urine, leading to night-time urination.

- Avoid excessive intake of fluid (take less than 3 liters of fluid per day). Instead of consuming a lot of fluid all at once, spread out intake of fluids over the day.

- Reduce fluid intake few hours before bedtime or going out.

- DO NOT take over-the-counter cold and sinus medications that contain decongestants or antihistamines. These medications can worsen symptoms or cause urinary retention.

- Change the timing of medications which increases volume of urine (e.g. diuretics).

- Keep warm and exercise regularly. Cold weather and lack of physical activity may worsen symptoms.

- Learn and perform pelvic strengthening exercises as they are useful to prevent urine leakage. Pelvic exercises strengthen the muscles of the pelvic floor which support the bladder and help in closing the

> **BPH with mild symptoms can be managed with watchful waiting and lifestyle changes and without medical treatment.**

sphincter. The exercises consist of repeatedly tightening and releasing the pelvic muscles.

- Bladder training focused on timed and complete voiding. Try to urinate at regular times.

- Treatment of constipation.

- Reduce stress. Nervousness and tension can lead to more frequent urination.

B. Medical Treatment

Medications are the most common and preferred way to control mild to moderate symptoms of BPH. Medications significantly reduce major symptoms in about two-thirds of treated men. There are two classes of drugs, alpha-blockers and anti-androgens (5-alpha-reductase inhibitors), for an enlarged prostate.

- **Alpha-blockers** (tamsulosin, alfuzosin, terazosin, and doxazosin) are prescription medicines that relax the muscles in and around the prostate, relieve urinary obstruction and allow urine to flow more easily. The most common side effects of alpha-blockers are light headedness, dizziness and fatigue.

- **5-alpha-reductase inhibitors** (finasteride and dutasteride) are medicines that can reduce the size of the prostate gland. These drugs increases urine flow rate, and decreases symptoms of BPH. They do not work as quickly as alpha-blockers (improvement is seen within six months of starting treatment) and generally work best on men with severe prostate enlargement. The most common side effects of 5-alpha-reductase inhibitors are problems with erection and ejaculation, decreased interest in sex and impotence.

Conservative medical treatment is preferred for mild to moderate symptoms of BPH. Surgery is best avoided.

- **Combination treatment:** An alpha blocker and an alpha-reductase inhibitor work differently and have an additive effect when given simultaneously. Therefore combination of both drugs leads to significantly greater improvement in the symptoms of BPH, than taking either drug by itself. Combination treatment is recommended in men with severe symptoms, large prostate and inadequate response to the highest dose of an alpha blocker.

C. Surgical Treatment

Surgical treatment is recommended in persons with:

- Bothersome, moderate to severe symptoms refractory to medical treatment.
- Acute urinary retention.
- Recurrent urinary tract infections.
- Recurrent or persistent blood in the urine.
- Kidney failure due to BPH.
- Bladder stones along with BPH.
- Increasing or significant post void residual urine in bladder.

Surgical treatment can be divided into two groups: surgical therapies and minimally invasive treatment. The standard surgical method is a transurethral resection of the prostate (TURP). Currently several newer methods are evolving in the surgical management of small to medium sized glands, which aim to achieve results comparable to TURP with less morbidity and cost.

Surgical Therapies

Specific surgical procedures commonly used are transurethral resection

---

Severe BPH symptoms, urinary retention, recurrent UTI and kidney failure indicate need for surgery.

---

of the prostate (TURP), transurethral incision of the prostate (TUIP) and open prostatectomy.

1. Transurethral Resection of the Prostate (TURP)

TURP remains the gold standard treatment of prostate surgery and is more successful than medication. It relieves urinary obstruction in at least 85% to 90% of cases, and the improvement is usually long-lasting. TURP is a minimally-invasive operation, performed by urologists to remove part of the prostate gland blocking urine flow. TURP does not require any skin incision or stitches, but requires hospitalization.

Before surgery

- Before the procedure, fitness of the person is ensured.

- The patient is asked to stop smoking as smoking increases the risk of getting a chest and wound infection, and can delay recovery.

- The patient is asked to discontinue blood-thinning medications (warfarin, aspirin and clopidogrel).

During the procedure

- TURP generally takes about 60 to 90 minutes.

- TURP is usually done using spinal anesthesia. Antibiotics are given to prevent infection.

- During TURP, an instrument (resectoscope) is inserted in the urethra through the tip of the penis to remove the prostate.

- The resectoscope has a light and camera for vision, an electrical loop to cut tissue and seal blood vessels, and a channel which carries irrigating fluid into the bladder.

- Prostate tissue removed during the procedure is sent to a laboratory for histopathological examination to exclude prostate cancer.

The most effective and popular surgical treatment of BPH is TURP.

After surgery

- The hospital stay is usually 2 to 3 days after TURP.
- Following surgery, a large triple lumen catheter is inserted through the tip of the penis (through the urethra) into the bladder.
- A bladder irrigation solution is attached to the catheter and the bladder is irrigated and drained continuously for about 12–24 hours.
- Bladder irrigation removes blood or blood clots that may result from the procedure.
- When the urine is free of significant bleeding or blood clots, the catheter is removed.

Advice after surgery

Following measures after TURP help in early recovery:

- Drink more fluids to flush out urine from the bladder.
- Avoid constipation and straining during defecation. Straining can result in increased bleeding. If constipation occurs, take a laxative for a few days.
- Do not start blood-thinning medications without advice of the doctor.
- Avoid heavy lifting or strenuous activity for 4-6 weeks.
- Avoid sexual activity for 4-6 weeks after surgery.
- Avoid alcohol, caffeine, and spicy foods.

Possible complications

- Immediate common complications are bleeding and urinary tract infection; while less common complications are TURP syndrome and problems from surgery.

TURP is done under spinal anesthesia without making the patient unconscious, thus, requiring a shorter hospital stay.

- Subsequent complications of TURP are narrowing (stricture) of the urethra, retrograde ejaculation, incontinence and impotence.

- Ejaculation of semen into the bladder (retrograde ejaculation) is a common sequel a of TURP, occurring in about 70% of cases. This does not affect sexual function or pleasure but causes infertility.

- Factors which can increase the risk of complications are obesity, smoking, alcohol abuse, malnutrition and diabetes.

After discharge from the hospital, contact the doctor if the patient has:

- Difficulty or inability to void.

- Severe pain which persists even after medications.

- Bleeding with large blood clots that block the catheter.

- Signs of infection, including fever or chills.

2. Transurethral Incision of the Prostate (TUIP)

Transurethral incision of the prostate (TUIP) is an alternative to TURP for men with smaller prostates or very poor health and therefore, not suitable for TURP.

The set-up for TUIP is similar to TURP, but rather than removing tissue from the prostate, two or more deep lengthwise incisions (cuts) are made in the prostate. The cuts widen the urethral passage, relieve pressure on the urethra and improve the flow of urine.

Benefits of TUIP are less blood loss, less surgery-related complications, shorter hospital stay and recovery time; and less risk of retrograde

---

Ejaculation of semen into bladder is a common complication of TURP leading to infertility (inability to father children).

---

ejaculation and urinary incontinence as compared to TURP. However, TUIP is less effective in providing symptom relief and/or symptoms return faster over a shorter period of time in some patients requiring a follow up treatment with TURP. TUIP is not the most effective method of treatment for a large-sized prostate.

3. Open Prostatectomy

Open prostatectomy is a type of surgery where an incision is made in the abdomen to remove the prostate. With availability of many effective and less invasive options, open prostatectomy is rarely used in the treatment of BPH.

An open prostatectomy is reserved only for very few men with severely enlarged prostates and in patients suffering from other problems that need simultaneous correction during surgery.

Minimally Invasive Treatments (MITs)

Minimally invasive methods are those that hurt the least. With modern technology and research, minimally invasive treatments are aimed at treating BPH through simpler procedures with less complications.

These treatment modalities generally use heat, laser, or electrovaporization to remove excess tissue from the prostate. All of these treatments use a transurethral approach (going up through the urethra in the penis).

Benefits of minimally invasive treatments are: shorter hospital stay, need for minimal anaesthesia, less risks and complications than standard prostate surgery, and shorter patient recovery times.

> **TUIP is an alternative to TURP for men with smaller prostates or high risk patients for whom TURP is not suitable.**

Disadvantages of these methods are: less effectiveness than standard TURP, more likely to need surgery again after 5 or 10 years, non availability of prostate tissue for histopathological examination (to exclude hidden prostate cancer) and fewer long-term studies for their safety and efficacy. Important additional drawback is that minimally invasive treatments (MITs) are not available in majority of developing countries and are currently more expensive.

Different minimally invasive treatments used in BPH are transurethral microwave thermotherapy (TUMT), transurethral needle ablation (TUNA), water-induced thermotherapy (WIT), prostate stents and transurethral laser therapy.

1. **Transurethral Microwave Thermotherapy (TUMT):** In this procedure, microwave heat is used to burn excess prostate tissue blocking urine flow.

2. **Transurethral Needle Ablation of the Prostate (TUNA):** In this procedure, radiofrequency energy is used to coagulate and necrose excess prostate tissue blocking urine flow.

3. **Water-Induced Thermotherapy (WIT):** In this technique, hot water causes heat-induced coagulation and necrosis of the excess prostate tissue.

4. **Prostatic Stents:** In this technique, a stent is placed within the narrowed area of the prostatic urethra. The stent keeps the channel open and allows easy urination. Stents are flexible, self-expanding titanium wire devices shaped like small springs or coils.

5. **Transurethral Laser Therapy:** In this technique, laser energy destroys the obstructing portions of the prostate by heating.

MIT benefits: less risks and shorter hospitalization; Concerns: cost effectiveness and long term safety.

When should a patient with BPH consult a doctor?

Patients with BPH should consult a doctor in case of:

- Complete inability to urinate.
- Pain or burning during urination, foul-smelling urine, or fever with chills.
- Blood in the urine.
- Loss of control of urination causing wetting of underclothes.

Prostatic stent is a safe and effective treatment when medications are ineffective & surgery is contraindicated.

Chapter 21
Drugs and Kidney Problems

Kidney damage due to different drugs is common.

Why is the kidney more vulnerable to drug toxicity compared to other organs of the body?

Two most important causes of damage to kidney due to drugs are:

1. Drug excretion by kidney: The kidney is a major organ involved in the removal of drugs and its metabolites. During the process of drug removal some drugs or its metabolites can damage the kidney.

2. High blood flow to kidney: Every minute 20% of total blood pumped by the heart (1200 ml blood) enters both kidneys for purification. Among all organs of the body, the kidney receives the highest amount of blood per kilogram weight of the organ. Because of the rich blood supply, harmful drugs and substances are delivered to the kidney in a large amount and in a short time. This can damage the kidney.

Principal drugs that damage the kidneys

1. Pain killers

For body ache, headache, joint pain and fever, various over the counter (OTC) medicines are available and these drugs are taken freely without doctor's prescription. These drugs are principally responsible for kidney damage.

What are NSAIDs? Which drugs belong to this group?

Non Steroidal Anti-Inflammatory Drugs (NSAIDs) are common medications used to reduce pain, fever and inflammation. These drugs

> **Pain killer drugs are a major cause of drug induced kidney damage.**

include aspirin, diclofenac, ibuprofen, indomethacin, ketoprofen, meloxicam, mefenamic acid, nimesulide, naproxen etc.

Do NSAIDs cause damage to kidneys?

NSAIDs are generally safe provided they are taken in correct doses under the supervision of a doctor. But it is important to remember that NSAIDs rank second to aminoglycosides as the most common cause of drug induced kidney damage.

When can NSAIDs damage kidneys?

Risk of NSAID induced kidney damage is high in cases of:

- Prolonged NSAID use taken in high dosages without supervision of a doctor.
- Prolonged use of a combination drug in a single pill (e.g. APC which contains aspirin, phenacetin and caffeine).
- NSAID use in the elderly, those with kidney failure, diabetes or dehydration.

Which pain killer is safe for kidney failure patients?

Paracetamol (acetaminophen) is a safer drug for pain compared to NSAIDs.

Many heart patients are prescribed lifelong aspirin. Can this damage the kidney?

Since a low dose of aspirin is advised for cardiac patients, it is safe.

Is kidney damage caused by NSAIDs reversible?

Yes and No.

Yes. When acute kidney damage is due to short term use of NSAIDs, it is usually reversible by stopping NSAID drugs and proper treatment.

Self-medication of common pain killer drugs can be dangerous.

No. Many elderly patients with joint pain need NSAIDs for a long period. When taken continuously in large doses for a long period (years) NSAID use can lead to slow and progressive kidney damage. This type of kidney damage is irreversible. Elderly patients, who need large doses of NSAIDs for a very long period, should take these medications under the guidance and supervision of a physician.

How does one diagnose slow but progressive kidney damage due to long term NSAIDs in the early stage?

Appearance of protein in urine is the first and only clue of kidney damage due to NSAIDs. When kidney function worsens creatinine level in blood rises.

How does one prevent kidney damage due to pain killers?

Simple measures to prevent kidney damage due to pain killers are:
- Avoid the use of NSAIDs in high risk persons.
- Avoid indiscriminate use of pain killers or OTC pain relievers.
- When NSAIDs are necessary for a long period, they should be taken strictly under the doctor's supervision.
- Limit dose and duration of treatment with NSAIDs.
- Avoid a combination of mixture of pain killers for a long period.
- Drink plenty of fluid daily. Adequate hydration is important to maintain proper blood supply to kidney and to avoid damage to kidney.

2. Aminoglycosides

Aminoglycosides are a group of antibiotics frequently used in practice and a common cause of kidney damage. Kidney damage occurs usually 7 - 10 days after the initiation of therapy. Diagnosis of this problem is often missed because volume of urine is unaltered.

> **Risk of drug induced kidney damage is high in patients with diabetes, kidney failure, dehydration or advanced age.**

The risk of aminoglycosides induced kidney damage is high in the elderly, dehydration, pre-existing kidney disease, potassium and magnesium deficiency, administration of large doses for prolonged periods, combination therapy with other drugs which can damage the kidney, sepsis, liver disease and congestive heart failure.

How does one prevent kidney damage due to aminoglycosides?

Measures to prevent the kidney damage due to aminoglycosides are:

- Cautious use of aminoglycosides in high risk persons. Correction or removal of the risk factors.
- Once-daily administration of aminoglycosides instead of divided dosage.
- Use of optimum dose and duration of aminoglycosides therapy.
- Dose modification in the presence of pre-existing kidney damage.
- Serial monitoring of serum creatinine every other day for early detection of kidney damage.

3. Radiocontrast injections

Radiographic contrast media (X-ray dyes) induced kidney damage is a common cause of acute kidney failure in hospitalized patients, and is usually reversible. The risk of contrast induced kidney damage is high in the presence of diabetes, dehydration, heart failure, pre-existing kidney damage, advanced age and concurrent use of drugs that can damage the kidney.

Different measures can prevent contrast induced kidney damage. Important measures are use of smallest dose of contrast, use of nonionic

For high risk patients, administer aminoglycosides cautiously & monitor serum creatinine serially to prevent kidney damage.

contrast agents, maintaining adequate hydration with IV fluids, and administration of sodium bicarbonate and acetylcysteine.

4. Other drugs

Other common drugs that can damage kidneys are certain antibiotics, anticancer therapy, antituberculosis drugs etc.

5. Other medicines

- The popular belief that all natural medicines (Aurvedic medicines, Chinese herbs etc.) and dietary supplements are harmless is wrong.

- Certain medicines of these groups contain heavy metals and toxic substances which can cause damage to the kidney.

- Use of certain medicines of these groups can be dangerous in patients with kidney failure.

- Certain drugs with high potassium content can be lethal in kidney failure.

It is a wrong belief that all natural medicines are always safe for the kidney.

Chapter 22
Nephrotic Syndrome

Nephrotic syndrome is a common kidney disease characterized by heavy loss of protein in urine, low blood protein levels, high cholesterol levels and swelling. This disease can occur at any age but is seen more frequently in children compared to adults. Nephrotic syndrome is characterized by its cycle of response to treatment, manifested by gradual tapering and discontinuation of medication, treatment free period of remission and frequent relapses causing swelling. As the cycle of recovery and recurrence repeats for a long period (years), this disease is a matter of worry for both the child and the family.

What is nephrotic syndrome?

The kidney works as a sieve (filter) in our body that removes waste products and extra water from blood and passes them out via the urine. The size of the holes of these filters is so small so that in normal circumstances proteins that are large in size do not pass into the urine.

In nephrotic syndrome the holes of these filters become large, so protein leaks into the urine. Because of the loss of protein in urine, the level of protein in the blood falls. Reduction of protein level in blood causes swelling (the medical term for the swelling seen in these patients is edema). The severity of edema varies depending on the amount of protein lost in the urine and reduction in protein level of blood. The kidney function (i.e., the ability to filter waste products or the glomerular filtration rate), per se, is normal in most patients with nephrotic syndrome.

Most important cause of recurrent swelling in children is nephrotic syndrome.

What causes nephrotic syndrome?

In over 90% of children the cause of nephrotic syndrome (called primary or idiopathic nephrotic syndrome) is not known. Primary Nephrotic Syndrome is caused by four pathological types: minimal change disease (MCD), focal segmental glomerulosclerosis (FSGS), membranous nephropathy and membranoproliferative glomerulonephritis (MPGN). Primary nephrotic syndrome is a "diagnosis of exclusion", i.e. they are diagnosed only after secondary causes have been excluded.

In less than 10 % of cases, nephrotic syndrome may be secondary to different conditions such as infection, drug exposure, malignancy, hereditary disorders or systemic diseases such as diabetes, systemic lupus erythematosus and amyloidosis.

Minimal change disease

The most common cause of nephrotic syndrome in children is minimal change disease (MCD). This disease occurs in 90 percent of cases of idiopathic nephrotic syndrome in young children (under age six) and in 65% of cases in older children.

In a typical child with minimal change disease, blood pressure is normal, red blood cells are absent in urine and the values of serum creatinine and complement 3 (C3) are normal. Of all the causes of nephrotic syndrome, minimal change disease is the least stubborn, as over 90% of the patients respond well to steroid therapy.

Symptoms of nephrotic syndrome

- Nephrotic syndrome can occur at any age but is most common between the ages of 2 to 8 years. It affects boys more often than girls.

Nephrotic syndrome commonly occurs in children between the ages of 2 to 8 years.

- The first sign of nephrotic syndrome in children is usually puffiness or swelling around the eyes and swelling of the face. Because of puffiness around the eyes, the patient is likely to consult an ophthalmologist (eye doctor) first.
- In nephrotic syndrome swelling of the eyes and the face is most noticeable in the morning and is less marked in the evening.
- With time, the swelling develops in the feet, hands, abdomen and all over the body and is associated with increase in weight.
- Swelling may occur after a respiratory tract infection and fever in many patients.
- Excluding swelling, the patient is usually well, active and does not seem sick.
- A decreased urine output compared to normal is common.
- Frothy urine and white stain on tiles due to albumin in urine may be a revealing feature.
- Red urine, breathlessness and high blood pressure are less common in nephrotic syndrome.

What are the complications of nephrotic syndrome?

Possible complications of nephrotic syndrome include an increased risk of developing infections, blood clots in the veins (deep vein thrombosis), malnutrition, anemia, heart disease due to high cholesterol and triglycerides, kidney failure and different treatment-related complications.

Diagnosis:

A. Basic laboratory tests

In patients with swelling the first step is to establish a diagnosis of

> The first sign of nephrotic syndrome in children is swelling around the eyes and swelling of the face.

nephrotic syndrome. Laboratory tests should confirm (1) heavy loss of protein in the urine, (2) low blood protein levels, and (3) high cholesterol levels.

1. Urine tests

- Urine examination is the first test used in the diagnosis of nephrotic syndrome. Normally, routine examination of urine will show negative or trace protein (albumin). The presence of 3+ or 4+ protein in a random urine sample is suggestive of nephrotic syndrome. Remember though that the presence of albumin in urine is not a specific diagnostic confirmation of nephrotic syndrome. It only suggests urinary loss of protein. Further investigations are necessary to determine the exact cause of urine protein loss.

- After starting treatment, urine is tested regularly to assess its response to treatment. The absence of protein in urine tests suggests a positive response to treatment. For self monitoring, protein in urine can be estimated by using a urine dipstick at home.

- In microscopic examination of urine, red blood cells and white blood cells are usually absent.

- In nephrotic syndrome, the loss of protein in urine is more than 3.5 grams in a day. The amount of protein lost in 24 hours can be estimated by a 24-hour urine collection or more conveniently by a spot urine protein/creatinine ratio. These tests provide precise measurements of the amount of protein lost and identify whether protein loss is mild, moderate or heavy. In addition to its diagnostic value, estimation of urine protein loss in 24 hours is useful for monitoring response to treatment.

Urine test is very important for diagnosis as well as monitoring of treatment of nephrotic syndrome.

---

2. Blood tests

- The characteristic findings of nephrotic syndrome that accompany the high urine protein levels are low blood albumin level (less than 3 g/dL) and elevated cholesterol (hypercholesterolemia) in blood tests.

- The value of serum creatinine is normal in nephrotic syndrome due to minimal change disease, but may be increased in patients with more severe kidney damage from other forms of nephrotic syndrome like focal segmental glomerulosclerosis. Serum creatinine is measured to assess overall kidney function.

- Complete blood count is a routine blood test performed in most of the patients.

B. Additional tests

Once the diagnosis of nephrotic syndrome has been established, additional tests are performed selectively. These tests determine whether the nephrotic syndrome is primary (idiopathic) or secondary to a systemic disorder; and to detect the presence of associated problems or complications.

1. Blood tests

- Blood sugar, serum electrolytes, calcium and phosphorus.
- Testing for HIV, hepatitis B and C and VDRL test.
- Complement studies (C3, C4) and ASO titer.
- Antinuclear antibody (ANA), anti–double-stranded DNA antibody, rheumatoid factor and cryoglobulins.

2. Radiological tests

- An ultrasound of the abdomen is performed to determine the size

---

Important diagnostic clues are loss of protein in urine and low protein, high cholesterol and normal creatinine in blood tests.

---

and shape of the kidney, and to detect mass, kidney stone, cyst or other obstruction or abnormality.

- X-ray of the chest is done to rule out infections.

3. Kidney biopsy

The kidney biopsy is the most important test used to determine the exact underlying type or cause of nephrotic syndrome. In a kidney biopsy, a small sample of kidney tissue is taken and examined in a laboratory. (for further information read Chapter 4).

Treatment

In nephrotic syndrome the goals of treatment are to relieve symptoms, correct urinary loss of protein, prevent and treat complications and protect the kidney. Treatment of this disease usually lasts for a long period (years).

1. Dietary advice

The dietary advice/restriction for a patient with swelling differs once the swelling disappears with effective treatment.

- **In a patient with swelling:** Restriction of dietary salt and avoidance of table salt as well as foods that are high in sodium content, so as to prevent fluid accumulation and edema. Restriction of fluid is usually not required.

  Patients receiving high doses of daily steroids should restrict salt intake even in the absence of swelling to decrease the risk of developing hypertension.

  For patients with swelling, adequate amounts of proteins should be provided to replace the urine protein loss and prevent malnutrition.

In patients with swelling, salt restriction is necessary but during symptom-free period avoid unnecessary dietary restrictions.

An adequate amount of calories and vitamins should also be provided to these patients.

- **In symptom- free patients:** The dietary advice during the symptom-free period is a normal healthy diet. Unnecessary dietary restrictions should be avoided. Avoid restriction of salt and fluid. Provide an adequate amount of proteins. Avoid moderately high protein diets to prevent kidney damage and restrict protein intake in the presence of kidney failure. Increase intake of fruits and vegetables. Reduce the intake of fat in diet to control blood cholesterol levels.

2. Drug therapy

A. Specific drug treatment

- **Steroid therapy:** Prednisolone (steroid) is the standard treatment for inducing remission in nephrotic syndrome. Most children respond to this drug. Swelling and protein in the urine disappear within 1-4 weeks (urine free of protein is labeled as a remission).

- **Alternate therapy:** A small group of children who do not respond to steroid treatment and continue to lose protein in their urine need further investigation such as a kidney biopsy. Alternate drugs used in such patients are levamisole, cyclophosphamide, cyclosporin, tacrolimus and mycophenylate mofetil (MMF). These alternate drugs are used along with steroid therapy and help to maintain remission when the dose of steroid is tapered.

B. Supportive drug treatment

- Diuretic drugs to increase urine output and reduce swelling. They should be used only under supervision by a doctor as excessive use may cause kidney failure.

Prednisolone (steroid) is the standard first line treatment of nephrotic syndrome.

Free!!! 200+ Paged Kidney Book in 35+ Languages
Visit: www.KidneyEducation.com

- Antihypertensive drugs such as ACE inhibitors and angiotensin II receptor blockers to control blood pressure and to reduce the urinary loss of protein.
- Antibiotics to treat infections (e.g. bacterial sepsis, peritonitis, pneumonia).
- Statins (simvastatin, atorvastatin, rosuvastatin) to reduce cholesterol and triglycerides and prevent the risk of heart and blood vessel problems.
- Supplement calcium, vitamin D and zinc.
- Rabeprazole, pantoprazole, omeprazole or ranitidine for protection against steroid induced stomach irritation.
- Albumin infusions are generally not used because their effects last only transiently.
- Blood thinners such as warfarin (Coumadin) or heparin, may be required to treat or prevent clot formation.

3. Treatment of underlying causes

Meticulous treatment of underlying causes of secondary nephrotic syndrome such as diabetic kidney disease, lupus kidney disease, amyloidosis etc. is important. Proper treatment of these disorders is necessary to control nephrotic syndrome.

4. General advice

- Nephrotic syndrome is a disease that lasts for several years. The patient and his/her family should be educated about the nature of the disease and its outcome; type of medication used and its side effects; and benefits of prevention and early treatment of the infection. It is

> **Infection is an important cause of recurrence of nephrotic syndrome, so it is essential to protect children against infection.**

important to emphasize that extra care is necessary during relapse when swelling is present, but during remission the patient should be treated as a normal child.

- The infection should be treated adequately before initiating steroid therapy in case of nephrotic syndrome.

- Children with nephrotic syndrome are prone to respiratory and other infections. Prevention, early detection and treatment of infection are essential in nephrotic syndrome because infection can lead to a relapse of controlled disease (even when the patient is receiving treatment).

- To prevent infection, the family and child should be trained to drink clean water, wash hands thoroughly and avoid crowded areas or contact with infectious patients.

- Routine immunization is advised when steroid course is completed.

5. Monitoring and follow up

- As nephrotic syndrome is likely to last for a long period (years), it is important to have regular follow ups with a doctor as advised. During the follow up the patient is evaluated by the doctor for loss of protein in urine, weight, blood pressure, height, side effect of medication and development of complications, if any.

- Patients should weigh themselves frequently and record it. Weight chart helps to monitor fluid gain or loss.

- The family should be taught to test urine for protein at home regularly and maintain a diary of all urine test results and dosage and the details of all medications. It helps in early detection of relapse and its prompt treatment subsequently.

> **As nephrotic syndrome lasts for years, regular urine tests and follow up with the doctor are crucial.**

Why and how is prednisolone given in nephrotic syndrome?

- The first drug used in the treatment of nephrotic syndrome is prednisolone (a steroid) that effectively corrects the disease and stops loss of protein in urine.

- The doctor decides on the dosage, duration and method of administration of prednisolone. The patient is advised to take this drug with food to avoid irritation of the stomach.

- In the first attack the drug is usually given for about 4 months, divided into three phases. The drug is given daily for 4 to 6 weeks initially, as a single dose on alternate mornings subsequently and finally the dose of prednisolone is gradually decreased and then discontinued. The treatment for relapse of nephrotic syndrome is different from the treatment given for the first attack.

- Within 1 to 4 weeks of the treatment the patient is symptom free and the leakage of protein in the urine stops. It is very important to complete the course as advised by the doctor to prevent frequent relapses. One must not make the mistake of discontinuing the treatment out of the fear of side effects of prednisolone.

What are the side effects of prednisolone (corticosteroids)?

Prednisolone is the most commonly used drug for the treatment of nephrotic syndrome. Because of the possibility of several side effects this drug should be taken strictly under medical supervision.

Short-term effects

Common short-term side effects are increase in appetite, weight gain, swelling of the face, stomach irritation causing abdominal pain, increased

> **Optimum steroid therapy is essential to control the disease, prevent frequent relapses and reduce side effects of steroid.**

susceptibility to infection, increased risk of diabetes and high blood pressure, irritability, acne and excessive growth of facial hair.

Long-term effects

Common long-term side effects are weight gain, stunted growth in children, thin skin, stretch marks on thighs, arms, and abdominal area, slow wound healing, development of cataracts, hyperlipidemia, bone problems (osteoporosis, avascular necrosis of the hip) and muscle weakness.

Why are corticosteroids used in the treatment of nephrotic syndrome in spite of multiple side effects?

Serious side effects of corticosteroids are known but at the same time untreated nephrotic syndrome has its potential dangers.

Nephrotic syndrome can cause severe swelling and low protein in the body. Untreated disease may cause numerous complications, such as increased risk of infections, hypovolemia, thromboembolism (blood clots may obstruct blood vessels and cause strokes, heart attacks, and lung disease), lipid abnormalities, malnutrition and anemia. Children with untreated nephrotic syndrome quite often die from infections.

With the use of corticosteroids in childhood nephrotic syndrome the mortality rate has been reduced to around 3%. The optimal dose and duration of corticosteroid therapy under proper medical supervision are most beneficial and least harmful. Majority of steroid effects disappear with time after the discontinuation of therapy.

In order to obtain potential benefits of the therapy and avoid life-threatening complications of the disease, the developement of some side effects of corticosteroid is unavoidable.

Steroids should be taken strictly under medical supervision to reduce the possibility of side effects.

In the nephrotic child, with initial steroid therapy swelling subsides and urine becomes protein free, but swelling of face is seen again during the third or fourth week of steroid therapy. Why?

Two independent effects of steroids are increased appetite leading to weight gain and redistribution of fat. These lead to a round or swollen face. Steroid induced moon-shaped face is seen during the third or fourth week of steroid therapy, which mimics swelling of the face due to nephrotic syndrome.

How does one differentiate swelling of the face due to nephrotic syndrome from steroid-induced moon-shaped face?

Swelling of nephrotic syndrome starts with puffiness or swelling around the eyes and the face. Later swelling develops in feet, hands and all over the body. Swelling of the face due to nephrotic syndrome is most noticeable in the morning, immediately after waking and is less noticeable in the evening.

Swelling due to steroids predominantly affects the face and abdomen (because of redistribution of fat), but arms and legs remain normal or thin. Steroid-induced swelling remains the same all throughout the day.

Different characteristics of distribution and time of its maximum appearance help in the differentiation of these two similar conditions. In certain patients, blood tests are needed to resolve the diagnostic dilemma. In patients with swelling, low serum protein/ albumin and high cholesterol indicate relapse while normal values of both tests suggest steroid effect.

Steroid therapy can increase appetite, weight and cause swelling of the face and abdomen.

Why is it important to differentiate between swelling of the face due to nephrotic syndrome and steroid side effects?

To determine precise treatment strategy in a patient, it is important to differentiate between swelling due to nephrotic syndrome and steroid side effects.

Swelling due to nephrotic syndrome needs an increase in steroid dose, modification in the method of its administration, and at times, addition of other specific drugs and temporary supplementation of water pills (diuretics).

Facial swelling due to steroids, on the other hand, is the proof of long term steroid intake, and one should neither worry that the disease is out of control nor reduce the dose of the steroid rapidly out of fear of the drug toxicity. For long term control of nephrotic syndrome, continuation of steroid therapy as per recommendation of the doctor is essential. Diuretics should not be used to treat steroid induced swollen face because it is ineffective and can be harmful.

What are the chances of recurrence of nephrotic syndrome in children? How frequently does relapse occur?

Chances of recurrence or relapse of nephrotic syndrome is as high as 50-75% in a nephrotic child. The frequency of relapse varies from patient to patient.

Which drugs are used when steroid is ineffective in the treatment of nephrotic syndrome?

When steroid is ineffective in the treatment of nephrotic syndrome, other specific drugs used are levamisole, cyclophosphamide, cyclosporine, tacrolimus and mycophenolate mofetil (MMF).

To plan optimum therapy, it is essential to differentiate between swelling due to disease and steroids.

What are the indications suggesting the need for kidney biopsy in children with nephrotic syndrome?

There is no need to do a kidney biopsy before starting steroid treatment in children with nephrotic syndrome. But kidney biopsy is indicated in the presence of:

- Absence or inadequate response to adequate doses of steroid treatment (steroid resistance).

- Frequently relapsing or steroid dependent nephrotic syndrome. In the latter case, withdrawal of steroids results in relapse (reappearance of protein in the urine) necessitating reinstitution and eventual maintenance of steroid therapy.

- Atypical features of childhood nephrotic syndrome such as onset in the first year of life, elevated blood pressure, persistent presence of red cells in urine, impaired kidney function and low blood C3 level.

Nephrotic syndrome of unknown origin in adults requires a kidney biopsy for diagnosis before initiating steroid therapy.

What is the prognosis of nephrotic syndrome and what is the expected time factor for its cure ?

The prognosis depends on the cause of nephrotic syndrome. The most common cause of nephrotic syndrome in children is minimal change disease which carries good prognosis. Majority of children with minimal change disease respond very well to steroids and there is no risk of developing chronic kidney failure.

A small proportion of children with nephrotic syndrome may not respond to steroid therapy and may require further evaluation (additional blood tests and kidney biopsy). These children with steroid resistant nephrotic

> **There is no risk of kidney failure in children with minimal change disease.**

syndrome need treatment with alternative drugs (levamisole, cyclophosphamide, cyclosporin, tacrolimus etc) and have a high risk of developing chronic kidney failure.

With proper treatment of nephrotic syndrome protein leak stops and the child becomes almost normal. In majority of children, relapse occurs for many years (throughout childhood). As the child grows, frequency of relapse decreases. Complete cure of nephrotic syndrome usually occurs between the age of 11 to 14 years. These children have an excellent prognosis and lead a normal life as adults.

When should a person with nephrotic syndrome consult a doctor?

The family of a child with nephrotic syndrome should immediately consult a doctor if he or she develops:

- Pain in the abdomen, fever, vomiting or diarrhea.
- Swelling, rapid unexplained weight gain, marked reduction in urine volume.
- Signs of illness, e.g. if he or she stops playing and is inactive.
- Persistent severe cough with fever or severe headache.
- Chicken pox or measles.

Nephrotic syndrome which lasts for years slowly disappears with age.

Chapter 23

Urinary Tract Infection in Children

Urinary tract infection (UTI) is a common problem in children with short term and long term health problems.

Why do urinary tract infections require urgent attention and immediate treatment in children compared to adults?

Children with urinary tract infection need immediate attention because:

- UTI is a common cause of fever in children and ranks third among the most common infections in children after respiratory tract infection and diarrhea.

- Inadequate and delayed treatment may cause permanent kidney damage. Recurrent UTI causes kidney scars that in the long term can lead to high blood pressure, poor kidney growth and even chronic kidney disease.

- Because of its variable presentation, diagnosis of UTI is often missed. A high index of vigilance and suspicion are necessary for its diagnosis.

- There is a high risk of recurrence.

What are the predisposing factors for urinary tract infections in children?

The following are common risk factors for UTI in children:

- Having a shorter urethra makes UTI more common in girls.

- Wiping from back to front (instead of front to back) after coming from the toilet.

- Structural abnormality of the urinary tract (e.g. posterior urethral valve).

Urinary tract infection is a common cause of fever in children.

- The presence of congenital urinary tract anomalies such as vesicoureteral reflux (condition with an abnormal backward flow of urine from the bladder up the ureters and toward the kidneys) and posterior urethral valve.

- Uncircumcised boys are more likely to develop UTI than circumcised boys.

- Stone in the urinary tract.

- Other causes: constipation, poor perineal hygiene, prolonged catheterization or family history of UTI.

Symptoms of Urinary Tract Infection

Older children can complain if they have problems with urination. Common symptoms of urinary tract infections are the same in older children as those in adults and are discussed in Chapter 18.

Younger children are unable to complain. Crying while voiding, difficulty or pain when voiding, foul smelling urine and frequent unexplained fever are common complaints of children with UTI. Young children with UTI may also have poor appetite, vomiting or diarrhea, poor weight gain or weight loss, irritability or no symptoms at all.

Diagnosis of Urinary Tract Infection

Investigations performed in children with urinary tract infections include:

1. Basic investigations in urinary tract infection

- Screening tests for UTI: Urine microscopy or dipstick tests. Further details are discussed in Chapter 18.

- Definitive diagnostic test for UTI: Urine culture and sensitivity (Urine CS) test for confirmation of diagnosis, identification of the specific

---

Common symptoms of UTI in children are recurrent fever, poor weight gain and urinary problems.

---

bacteria causing infection and selection of the most appropriate antibiotic for treatment.

• Blood tests: Hemoglobin, total and differential white cell count, blood urea, serum creatinine, blood sugar and C reactive protein.

2. Investigations for diagnosis of risk factors of urinary tract infection

• Radiological tests to detect underlying abnormalities: Ultrasound of kidney and urinary bladder (KUB), X-rays of the abdomen, Voiding Cystourethrogram (VCUG), CT scan or MRI of the abdomen and Intravenous Urography (IVU).

• Tests to detect scarring of kidney: A dimercaptosuccinic acid (DMSA) kidney scan is the best method for detecting kidney scarring. DMSA scan should be done preferably 3 to 6 months after an episode of UTI.

• Urodynamic studies to assess bladder function.

What is a voiding cystourethrogram? When and how is it done?

• Voiding cystourethrogram or VCUG (previously known as Micturating cystourethrogram or MCU) is a very important diagnostic X-ray test for children with urinary tract infection and vesicoureteral reflux (VUR). VCUG test is the gold standard for the diagnosis of vesicoureteral reflux and its severity (grading), and detection of abnormalities of the urinary bladder and urethra. It should be done for every child below 2 years after the first episode of UTI.

• VCUG should be done after treating UTI, usually after the first week of diagnosis.

Most important tests to diagnose predisposing factors for UTI are ultrasound, VCUG and IVU.

- In this test the urinary bladder is filled to its capacity with contrast (radio opaque iodine containing dye fluid which can be seen on X-ray films) through a catheter under strict aseptic precautions and usually under antibiotic cover.

- A series of X-ray images are taken before and at timed intervals during voiding. This test provides a comprehensive view of the structure and the function of the bladder and urethra.

- VCUG can detect urine flow from the bladder backwards into the ureters or kidneys, known as vesicoureteral reflux.

- VCUG is also used to detect the presence of a posterior urethral valve in male infants.

Prevention of Urinary Tract Infection

1. Increasing fluid intake dilutes urine and helps in flushing out bacteria from the urinary bladder and urinary tract.

2. Children should urinate every two to three hours. Holding urine in the bladder for a long period of time provides opportunity for bacteria to grow.

3. Keep genital area of children clean. Wipe child from front to back (not back to front) after toilet. This habit prevents bacteria in the anal region from spreading to the urethra.

4. Frequently change diapers to prevent prolonged contact of stool with the genital area.

5. Children should be made to wear only cotton undergarments to allow air circulation. Avoid tight-fitting pants and nylon underwear.

6. Avoid giving bubble baths.

VCUG is the most reliable X-ray test used in children with UTI to detect vesicoureteral reflux and posterior urethral valve.

---

7. For the uncircumcised boy, the foreskin of his penis should be washed regularly.

8. In children with VUR, recommend double or triple voiding (passing of urine) to prevent residual urine.

9. A low dose daily antibiotic for long-term as a preventive (prophylactic) measure is recommended for some children who are prone to chronic UTI.

Treatment of Urinary Tract Infection

General measures

All preventive measures for urinary tract infection should be followed.

- A child with UTI should be advised to drink more water. Sick hospitalized children need intravenous fluid therapy.

- Appropriate medications should be given for fever.

- Urinalysis and urine culture and sensitivity should be done after completion of treatment to ensure that infection is controlled adequately. Regular follow up with urine tests is necessary for all children to confirm that there is no recurrence of infection.

- Ultrasound and other appropriate investigations should be done for all children with UTI.

Specific treatment

- In children, UTI should be treated with antibiotics without delay to protect the developing kidneys.

- Urine culture should be sent before initiating treatment to identify causative bacteria and properly select antibiotics.

- A child needs hospitalization and intravenous antibiotics if he/ she

---

Inadequate and delayed treatment of UTI in children can cause irreversible kidney damage.

---

has high grade fever, vomiting, severe flank pain and is unable to take medicine by mouth.

- Oral antibiotics may be given to children more than 3 to 6 months of age who are able to take oral medications.

- It is important that children complete a full course of prescribed antibiotics, even if the child no longer has symptoms of UTI.

Recurrent urinary tract infection

Children with recurrent, symptomatic UTI need additional tests such as ultrasound, VCUG and at times DMSA scan to identify the underlying cause. Three important treatable problems for recurrent UTI are VUR, the posterior urethral valves and kidney stones. According to the underlying cause, specific medical treatment followed by preventive measures and long term preventive antibiotics therapy is planned. In some children surgical treatment is planned jointly by the nephrologist and urologist.

Posterior Urethral Valves

Posterior urethral valve (PUV) is a congenital abnormality of the urethra which occurs in boys. It is the most common cause of obstruction of the lower urinary tract in boys.

Basic problem and its importance: Folds of tissue within the urethra lead to incomplete or intermittent blockage to the normal flow of urine in PUV. A blockage to the urine flow through the urethra causes back pressure on the urinary bladder. The size of the bladder increases considerably and its muscle wall becomes very thick.

A very large urinary bladder with elevated bladder pressure leads to an

Send urine for CS before initiating therapy to identify causative bacteria & select appropriate antibiotics.

increase in pressure which is felt by the ureters and kidney. This results in dilatation (widening) of the ureters and the pelvocalyceal (drainage) system of the kidneys. Such dilatation, if not diagnosed and treated timely, can lead to chronic kidney disease (CKD) in the long term. About 25% to 30% children born with PUV are likely to suffer from end stage kidney disease (ESKD). PUV is therefore a significant cause of morbidity and mortality in infants and children.

Symptoms: Common symptoms of posterior urethral valves are weak urine stream, dribbling of urine, difficulty or straining to when voiding , bedwetting, fullness of the lower part of the abdomen (supra pubic region) due to a palpable urinary bladder and urinary tract infection.

Diagnosis: Ultrasound before birth (antenatal) or after birth in a male child provides the first clue for the diagnosis of PUV. Confirmation of the diagnosis of PUV requires the VCUG test that is carried out in the immediate postnatal period.

Treatment: Surgeons (urologists) and kidney specialists (nephrologists) jointly treat PUV. The first treatment for immediate improvement is to insert a tube into the urinary bladder (usually through the urethra and occasionally directly through the abdominal wall - suprapubic catheter) to drain urine continuously. Simultaneous supportive measures such as treatment of infection, anemia and kidney failure; and correction of malnutrition, fluid and electrolyte abnormalities help in the improvement of the general condition.

Definitive treatment of PUV is surgical removal of the valve with the use of an endoscope. All children need regular lifelong follow up with a nephrologist subsequently because of the risk of UTI, problems of growth, electrolyte abnormalities, anemia, high blood pressure and chronic kidney disease.

PUV causes obstruction of the lower urinary tract in boys leading to CKD if not treated in time.

Vesicoureteral Reflux (VUR)

Vesicoureteral reflux (VUR) is "backward flow of urine from bladder into ureter".

Why is it important to know about vesicoureteral reflux?

VUR is present in about 30 to 40 % of children with UTI associated with fever. In many children VUR may cause scarring and damage to the kidneys. Kidney scarring for a long period may cause high blood pressure, toxemia of pregnancy in young females, chronic kidney disease and, in a few patients, end stage kidney disease. VUR is more common in family members of a person with VUR and affects girls more frequently.

What is vesicoureteral reflux and why does it occur?

VUR is a condition with an abnormal backward flow (reflux) of urine from the bladder toward the ureters and possibly up to the kidneys. This can happen on either one or both sides.

Urine formed in kidneys flows down to the urinary bladder through the ureters. Urine normally flows in one direction, down the ureters and into the urinary bladder.

During urination and when the urinary bladder is filled with urine, a valve between the bladder and ureter is responsible for the prevention of back flow of urine into the ureters. VUR is caused by a defect in the mechanism of this valve.

VUR can be graded from mild to severe (Grade I to V) based on the severity of back flow of urine from the urinary bladder to the ureters and kidneys.

VUR is very common in children with UTI and carries the risk of hypertension and CKD.

Vesicoureteral Reflux

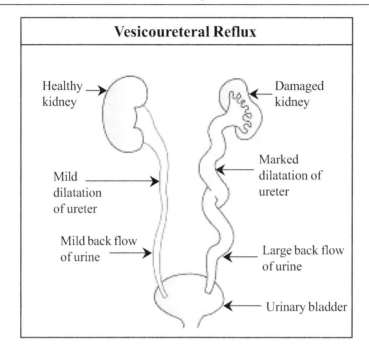

Healthy kidney

Damaged kidney

Mild dilatation of ureter

Marked dilatation of ureter

Mild back flow of urine

Large back flow of urine

Urinary bladder

What causes vesicoureteral reflux?

There are two types of VUR: primary VUR and secondary VUR. Primary VUR is the most common type of VUR and is present at birth. Secondary VUR can occur at any age. It commonly occurs due to obstruction or malfunction in the bladder or urethra with bladder infection.

What are the symptoms of vesicoureteral reflux?

There are no specific signs and symptoms of VUR. But frequent and recurrent urinary tract infection (UTI) is the most common presentation of VUR. In older children with untreated severe vesicoureteral reflux, signs and symptoms are apparent because of complications such as high blood pressure, protein in urine or kidney failure.

How is vesicoureteral reflux (VUR) diagnosed?

Investigations performed in children with suspected VUR are:

1. Basic diagnostic test for VUR

- Voiding cystourethrogram - VCUG is the gold standard for the diagnosis of vesicoureteral reflux and its severity (grading).

- Vesicoureteral reflux is graded according to the degree of reflux. The grade of VUR indicates how much urine is flowing backward into the ureters and kidneys. Grading is important in determining prognosis and most appropriate therapy for a given patient.

- In the mild form of VUR, urine refluxes only to the ureter (Grade I and II). In the most severe form of VUR there is massive reflux of urine, with marked tortuosity and dilatation of the ureter and severe kidney swelling (Grade V).

2. Additional investigations in VUR

- Urine test and urine culture: used to detect a urinary tract infection.

- Blood tests: basic tests usually performed are hemoglobin, white blood cells and serum creatinine. Serum creatinine can be used as a measure of kidney function.

- Kidney and bladder ultrasound: to find out the size and shape of the kidneys and to detect scars, kidney stones, obstruction or other abnormalities. It cannot detect reflux.

- DMSA kidney scan: this is the best method for detecting kidney scarring.

How is vesicoureteral reflux treated?

It is important to treat VUR to prevent possible infections and kidney damage. The management of vesicoureteral reflux depends on the grade of reflux, age of children and symptoms. There are three treatment options for VUR, : antibiotics, surgery and endoscopic treatment. The

---

With regular antibiotics for a long term (years), low-grade reflux resolves without surgery.

---

most common first-line treatment of VUR is the use of antibiotics to prevent UTI. Surgery and endoscopic treatment is reserved for severe VUR or in those cases where antibiotics have not been effective.

Mild VUR: Mild VUR will resolve completely on its own by the time a child is 5 to 6 years old. Children with mild VUR are less likely to need surgery. In such patients, a low dosage of antibiotics is given once or twice a day for a prolonged period of time to prevent UTI. This is called antibiotic prophylaxis. Antibiotic prophylaxis is usually given until the patient is 5 years of age. Remember that antibiotics per se do not correct VUR. Nitrofurantoin and cotrimoxazole are preferred drugs for antibiotic prophylaxis.

All children with VUR should follow general preventive measures for UTI (discussed above) and regular frequent and double voiding. Periodic urine tests are needed to detect UTI. VCUG and ultrasound are repeated yearly to determine if reflux has subsided.

Severe VUR: The severe form of VUR is less likely to resolve on its own. Children with the severe form of VUR require surgery or endoscopic treatment. Correction of reflux by open surgery (ureteral reimplantation or ureteroneocystostomy) prevents the backflow of urine. The main advantage of surgery is its high success rate (88-99%).

Endoscopic treatment is a second effective treatment modality for the severe form of VUR. The benefits of endoscopic technique are that it can be performed in an outpatient setting, takes just 15 minutes, has fewer risks and does not require any incision. Endoscopic treatment is done under general anesthesia. In this method with the help of an endoscope (lighted tube) a special bulking material (e.g. Dextranomer/ hyaluronic acid copolymer - Deflux) is injected into the area where the ureter enters the urinary bladder. Injection of the bulking material

---

Surgery and endoscopic treatment are indicated in severe VUR or when antibiotics are not successful.

---

increases the resistance at the entry of the ureter and prevents urine from flowing back into the ureter. The success rate for resolution of reflux with this method is about 85 to 90%. Endoscopic treatment is a convenient treatment option in the earlier stage of VUR as it avoids long term use of antibiotics and the stress of living with VUR for years.

Follow-up: All children with VUR should be regularly monitored with measurement of height, weight, blood pressure, urine analysis and other tests as recommended by his/her doctor.

When should a patient with UTI consult a doctor?

For children with urinary tract infection the doctor should immediately be consulted in case of:

- Persistent fever, chills, pain or burning during urination, foul-smelling urine or blood in the urine.
- Nausea or vomiting which prevents intake of fluid and medication.
- Dehydration due to poor fluid intake or vomiting.
- Pain in the lower back or abdomen.
- Irritability, poor appetite, failure to thrive or child is unwell.

> **Regular follow up is advised in VUR to assess blood pressure, growth, recurrence of UTI and damage to the kidneys.**

Bedwetting or involuntary passing of urine during sleep is quite common in children. In most cases it spontaneously resolves without any treatment as children grow up. However it is still worrisome for the children and their families because it causes inconvenience and embarrassment. It is not due to kidney disease, laziness or naughtiness of children.

What percentage of children suffers from bedwetting and at what age does it normally stop?

Bedwetting is common especially under the age of 6 years. At the age of 5 years, bedwetting occurs in about 15 to 20 % of children. With increasing age, there is a proportionate decrease in the prevalence of bedwetting: 5% at 10 years, 2% at 15 years, and less than 1% in adults.

Which children are more likely to suffer from bedwetting ?

- Children whose parents have had the same problem in childhood.
- Those with delayed neurological development which reduces the child's ability to recognize a full bladder.
- Children with deep sleep.
- Boys are affected more often than girls.
- Increased psychological or physical stress may be the trigger.
- In a very small percentage of children (2%-3%), medical problems such as urinary tract infection, diabetes, kidney failure, pin worms, constipation, small bladder, abnormalities in the spinal cord or defect in the urethral valves in boys, are responsible.

Bedwetting at night is a common problem in young children, but it is not a disease.

When and which investigations are performed for bedwetting children?

Investigations are performed only in selected children when medical or structural problems are suspected. The most frequently performed tests are urine tests, blood glucose, X-rays of spine and ultrasound examination or other imaging tests of the kidneys or bladder.

Treatment

Bedwetting is completely involuntary and is not done intentionally. Children should be reassured that bedwetting will stop or be cured over time. They should not be scolded or punished.

Initial treatment for bedwetting includes education, motivational therapy and change in habits of fluid intake and voiding. If bedwetting does not improve with these measures, bedwetting alarms or medications may be tried.

1. Education and motivational therapy

- The child must be thoroughly educated about bedwetting.
- Bedwetting is not the fault of the children so they should not be blamed or admonished about bedwetting.
- Take care that no one teases the child for bedwetting. It is important to reduce the stress the child suffers due to bedwetting. The child's family should be supportive and the child should be reassured that the problem is temporary and it is sure to be corrected.
- Use training pants instead of diapers.
- Ensure easy access to the toilet at night by properly arranging night lamps.

> **With increasing age, a sympathetic approach and motivation will cure the problem of bedwetting.**

- Keep an extra pair of pajamas, bed sheet and a towel handy, so that the child can change bed linens and soiled clothing conveniently if he wakes up due to bedwetting.

- Cover the mattress with plastic to avoid damage to the mattress.

- Place a large towel underneath the bed sheet for extra absorption.

- Encourage daily bath in the morning so that there is no urine smell.

- Praise and reward your child for a dry night. Even a small gift is an encouragement for a child.

- Constipation must not be neglected, it should be treated.

2. Limit fluid intake

- Limit the amount of fluid the child drinks two to three hours before bedtime, but ensure adequate fluid intake during the day.

- Avoid caffeine (tea, coffee), carbonated drinks (cola) and chocolate in the evening. They can increase the need to urinate and aggravate bedwetting.

3. Advice on voiding habits

- Encourage double voiding before bed. First voiding at routine bedtime and second voiding just before falling asleep.

- Make it a habit to use the toilet at regular intervals throughout the day.

- Wake the child up about three hours after he falls asleep every night to void urine. If necessary, use an alarm.

- By determining the most likely time of bedwetting, the waking time can be adjusted.

Limiting fluid intake before bedtime and discipline in voiding habits are the most important measures to prevent bedwetting.

---

4. Bedwetting alarms

- The use of bedwetting or moisture alarms is the most effective method for controlling bedwetting and is generally reserved for children older than 7 years of age.

- In this alarm a sensor is attached to the child's underwear. When the child voids in bed, the device senses the first drops of urine, rings and wakes up the child. The woken up child can control his urine until he reaches the toilet.

- The alarm helps in training the child to wake up just in time before the bedwetting problem.

5. Bladder training exercises

- Many children with bedwetting problems have small bladders. The goal of bladder training is to increase the capacity of the bladder.

- During day time children are asked to drink a large quantity of water and told to hold back urine in spite of the urge to pass urine.

- With practice, a child can hold urine for longer periods of time. This will strengthen the bladder muscles and will increase bladder capacity.

6. Drug therapy

Medications are used as a last resort to stop bedwetting and are generally used only in children over seven years old. These are effective, but do not "cure" bedwetting. These provide a stopgap measure and are best used on a temporary basis. Bedwetting usually recurs when the medication is stopped. Permanent cure is more likely with bedwetting alarms than with medications.

Bedwetting alarms and drug therapy are generally adopted for children older than 7 years of age.

A. Desmopressin Acetate (DDAVP): Desmopressin tablets are available in the market and prescribed when other methods are unsuccessful. This drug reduces the amount of urine produced at night and is useful only in those children who produce a large volume of urine. While the child is on this medication, remember to reduce evening fluid intake to avoid water intoxication. This drug is usually given before bedtime and should be avoided at night when the child has, for any reason, drunk a lot of fluids.

Although this drug is very effective and has few side effects, its use is limited because of its prohibitive cost.

B. Imipramine: Imipramine (a tricyclic antidepressant) has a relaxing effect on the bladder and tightens the sphincter and thereby increases the capacity of the bladder to hold urine. This drug is usually used for about 3-6 months. Because of its rapid effect, the drug is taken one hour before bedtime. This drug is highly effective, but because of frequent side effects it is used selectively. Side effects may include nausea, vomiting, weakness, confusion, insomnia, anxiety, palpitations, blurred vision, dry mouth and constipation.

C. Oxybutynin: Oxybutynin (an anticholinergic drug) is useful for daytime bedwetting. This drug reduces bladder contractions and increases bladder capacity. Side effects may include dry mouth, facial flushing and constipation.

When should one consult a doctor for children with bedwetting problems?

The family of a child with bedwetting should immediately consult a doctor if the child:

- Has a day time bedwetting problem.
- Continues bedwetting after the age of seven or eight years.

For bedwetting, drug therapy is an effective stopgap measure for short term benefit but it is not curative.

- Starts bedwetting again after at least six months of a dry period.
- Loses control in defecation or passing stools.
- Has fever, pain, burning and frequent urination, unusual thirst, and swelling of the face and feet.
- Has poor stream of urine, difficulty in voiding or needs to strain when urinating.

In cases of daytime bedwetting accompanied by fever, burning in urination or bowel difficulties, consult your doctor immediately.

Chapter 25

Diet in Chronic Kidney Disease

The major role of the kidneys is to remove waste products and purify blood. Besides this, the kidney plays an important role in removing extra water, minerals and chemicals; it also regulates water and minerals like sodium, potassium, calcium, phosphorus and bicarbonate in the body.

In patients suffering from chronic kidney disease (CKD), regulation of fluids and electrolytes may be deranged. Because of this reason even normal intake of water, common salt or potassium can cause serious disturbances in fluid and electrolyte balance.

To reduce the burden on the kidney with impaired function and to avoid disturbances in fluid and electrolyte balance, patients with chronic kidney disease should modify their diet as per the guidance of the doctor and the dietitian. There is no fixed diet for CKD patients. Each patient is given a different dietary advice depending on clinical status, the stage of kidney failure and other medical problems. Dietary advice needs to be altered for the same patient at different times.

The goals of dietary therapy in CKD patients are to:

1. Slow down the progression of chronic kidney disease and to postpone the need for dialysis.
2. Reduce the toxic effects of excess urea in the blood.
3. Maintain optimal nutritional status and prevent the loss of lean body mass.
4. Reduce the risk of fluid and electrolyte disturbances.
5. Reduce the risk of cardiovascular disease.

General principles of dietary therapy in CKD patients are:

- Restrict protein intake to <0.8 gm/kg of body weight/day for patients not on dialysis. Patients already on dialysis require an increased amount of protein (1.0 -1.2 gm/kg body weight/day) to replace protein that may be lost during the procedure.

- Supply adequate carbohydrates to provide energy.
- Supply a moderate amount of fats. Cut down the intake of butter, ghee and oil.
- Limit the intake of fluid and water in case of swelling (edema).
- Restrict the amount of sodium, potassium and phosphorus in the diet.
- Supply vitamins and trace elements in adequate amounts. A high fiber diet is recommended.

Details of selection and modification in diet of patients with CKD are as follows:

1. High Calorie Intake

The body needs calories for daily activities and to maintain temperature, growth and adequate body weight. Calories are supplied chiefly by carbohydrates and fats. The usual caloric requirement of CKD patients is 35 - 40 kcal/kg body weight per day. If caloric intake is inadequate, the body utilizes protein to provide calories. This breakdown of protein can lead to harmful effects such as malnutrition and a greater production of waste products. It is thus essential to provide an adequate amount of calories to CKD patients. It is important to calculate the caloric requirement according to a patient's ideal body weight, and not current weight.

Carbohydrates

Carbohydrates are the primary source of calories for the body. Carbohydrates are found in wheat, cereals, rice, potatoes, fruits and vegetables, sugar, honey, cookies, cakes, sweets and drinks. Diabetics and obese patients need to limit the amount of carbohydrates. It is best to use complex carbohydrates from cereals like whole wheat and unpolished rice which would also provide fiber. These should form a large portion of the carbohydrates in the diet. All other simple sugar containing substances should form not more than 20% of the total carbohydrate intake, especially in diabetic patients. Non-diabetic patients may replace calories from protein with carbohydrates in the form of fruits, pies, cakes, cookies, jelly or honey as long as desserts with chocolate, nuts, or bananas are limited.

Fats

Fats are an important source of calories for the body and provide two times more calories than carbohydrates or proteins. Unsaturated or "good" fats like olive oil, peanut oil, canola oil, safflower oil, sunflower oil, fish and nuts are better than saturated or "bad" fats such as red meat, poultry, whole milk, butter, ghee, cheese, coconut and lard. Patients with CKD should reduce their intake of saturated fats and cholesterol, as these can cause heart disease.

Among the unsaturated fats it is important to pay attention to the proportion of monounsaturated and polyunsaturated fats. Excessive amounts of omega-6 polyunsaturated fatty acids (PUFA) and a very high omega-6/omega-3 ratio is harmful while low omega-6/omega-3 ratio exerts beneficial effects. Mixtures of vegetable oil rather than single oil usage will achieve this purpose. Trans fat containing substances like potato chips, doughnuts, commercially prepared cookies and cakes are potentially harmful and should be avoided.

2. Restrict Protein Intake

Protein is essential for the repair and maintenance of body tissues. It also helps in healing of wounds and fighting against infection. Protein restriction (< 0.8 gm/kg body weight/day) is recommended for CKD patients not on dialysis to reduce the rate of decline in kidney function and delay the need for dialysis and kidney transplantation. Severe protein restriction should be avoided however because of the risk of malnutrition. Poor appetite is common in CKD patients. Poor appetite and strict protein restriction together can lead to poor nutrition, weight loss, lack of energy and reduction in body resistance, which increase the risk of death. Proteins with high biologic value such as animal protein (meat, poultry and fish), eggs and tofu are preferred. High-protein diets (e.g. Atkins diet) should be avoided in CKD patients. Likewise, the use of protein supplements and drugs such as creatine used for muscle development are best avoided unless approved by a physician or dietitian. However, once a patient is on dialysis, protein intake should be increased to 1.0 – 1.2 gm/kg body weight/day to replace the proteins lost during the procedure.

3. Fluid Intake

Why must patients with CKD take precautions regarding fluid intake?

The kidneys play a major role in maintaining the proper amount of water in the body by removing excess fluid as urine. In patients with CKD, as the kidney function worsens, the volume of urine usually decreases.

Reduced urine output leads to fluid retention in the body causing puffiness of the face, swelling of the legs and hands and high blood pressure. Accumulation of fluid in the lungs (a condition called pulmonary congestion or edema) causes shortness of breath and difficulty in breathing. If this is not controlled, it can be life threatening.

What are the clues that suggest excess water in the body?

Excess water in the body is called fluid overload. Leg swelling (edema), ascites (accumulation of fluid in the abdominal cavity), shortness of breath, and weight gain in a short period are the clues that suggest fluid overload.

What precautions must CKD patients take to control fluid intake?

To avoid fluid overload or deficit, the volume of fluid should be recorded and followed as per the recommendation of the doctor. The volume of fluid permitted may vary for each CKD patient and is calculated on the basis of urine output and fluid status of each patient.

How much fluid is a chronic kidney disease patient advised to take?

- In patients without edema and with adequate urine output, unrestricted water and fluid intake is permitted. It is a common misconception that patients with kidney disease should take large amounts of fluid to protect the kidney. The amount of fluid allowed is dependent on the clinical status and kidney function of the patient.

- Patients with edema and reduced urine output are instructed to restrict fluid intake. To reduce swelling, fluid intake in 24hours should be less than the volume of urine produced per day.

- In order to avoid fluid overload or deficit in patients without edema, the allowable volume of fluid per day = urine volume of previous day plus 500 ml. The additional 500 ml of fluid approximately makes up for the fluids lost through perspiration and breathing.

Why must CKD patients maintain a record of their daily weights?

Patients should keep a record of their daily weight to monitor fluid volume in the body and to detect fluid gain or loss. The body weight remains constant when the instructions regarding fluid intake are followed strictly. Sudden weight gain indicates fluid overload due to increase in fluid intake. Weight gain warns the patients about the need for more meticulous fluid restriction. Weight loss usually occurs as a combined effect of restriction of fluid and a response to diuretics.

Useful Tips to Reduce Fluid Intake :

It is difficult to restrict fluid intake, but these tips will help you:

1. Weigh yourself at the same time every day and adjust fluid intake accordingly.

2. The doctor advises you on how much fluid consumption is permitted in a day. Calculate accordingly and take the measured volume of fluid everyday. Remember that fluid intake includes not only water but also tea, coffee, milk, juice, ice cream, cold drinks, soup, and other foods with a high water content such as watermelon, grapes, lettuce, tomatoes, celery, gravy, gelatin, and frozen treats like popsicles.

2. Reduce salty, spicy and fried food in your diet as they increase thirst, leading to a greater consumption of fluids.

3. Drink only when you are thirsty. Do not drink as a habit or because everyone is drinking.

4. When you are thirsty, take only a small amount of water or try ice. Take a small ice cube and suck it. Ice stays longer in the mouth than liquid, so it is more satisfying than the same amount of water. Do not forget to account for ice as consumed fluid. For easy calculation, freeze the allotted amount of water into an ice tray.

5. To take care of dryness of the mouth, one can gargle with water without drinking it. Dryness of mouth can be reduced by chewing gums, sucking hard candy, lemon wedge or mints and the use of mouthwash to moisten the mouth.

6. Always use a small sized cup and glass for your beverages to limit fluid intake.

7. Take medicines after meals when you are taking water to avoid extra water consumption for medicine.

8. A patient must keep himself busy with work. A patient who has little to occupy himself feels the desire to drink water more often.

9. High blood sugar in diabetic patients can increase thirst. A stringent control of blood sugar is essential to reduce thirst.

10. Since hot weather increases one's thirst, any measure taken to live in cooler comfort is desirable and recommended.

How does one measure and consume the prescribed amount of fluid per day?

*   Fill a container with water, equal to the exact amount of fluid prescribed by the doctor for daily intake.

*   The patient must bear in mind that no more than that amount of fluid intake is permitted for the day.

*   Each time the patient consumes a certain amount of fluid, the same amount of water should be removed from the water container and discarded.

*   When the container has no more water, the patient will have consumed his quota of fluid for the day and should not drink anymore.

*   It is advisable to distribute total fluid intake evenly throughout the day to avoid the need for additional fluid.

*   Repeated daily, this method, if followed, effectively delivers the prescribed amount of fluid per day and prevents excessive fluid intake.

4. Salt (Sodium) Restriction in Diet

Why is a low sodium diet advised for patients with CKD?

Sodium in our diet is important for the body to maintain blood volume and to control blood pressure. Our kidneys play an important role in the regulation of sodium. In patients with CKD, the kidneys cannot remove excess sodium and fluid from the body so sodium and water build up in the body. An increased amount of sodium in the body leads to increased thirst, swelling, shortness of breath and increase in blood pressure. To prevent or reduce these problems, patients with CKD must restrict sodium intake in their diet.

What is the difference between sodium and salt?

The words sodium and salt are commonly used as synonyms. Common salt (table salt) is sodium chloride and contains 40% sodium. Salt is the principle source of sodium in our diet. But salt is not the only source of sodium. There are quite a few other sodium compounds in our food, such as:

- Sodium alginate: Used in ice-cream and chocolate milk
- Sodium bicarbonate: Used as baking powder and soda
- Sodium benzoate: Used as a preservative in sauce
- Sodium citrate: Used to enhance flavor of gelatin, desserts and beverages
- Sodium nitrate: Used in preserving and coloring processed meat
- Sodium saccharide: Used as artificial sweetener
- Sodium sulfite: Used to prevent discoloration of dried fruits

The above mentioned compounds contain sodium but are not salty in taste. Sodium is hidden in these compounds.

How much salt should one take?

A typical daily intake of salt is about 10 to 15 grams (4-6 grams of sodium) per day. Patients with CKD should take salt according to the recommendation of the doctor. CKD patients with edema (swelling) and high blood pressure are usually advised to take less than 2 grams of sodium per day.

Which foods contain high amounts of sodium?

Foods high in sodium include:

1. Table salt (common salt), baking powder
2. Processed foods like canned foods, fast foods and "deli" meats

3.   Readymade sauces

4.   Seasonings and condiments such as fish sauce and soy sauce

5.   Baked food items like biscuits, cakes, pizza and breads

6.   Wafers, chips, popcorn, salted groundnuts, salted dry fruits like cashew nuts and pistachios

7.   Commercial salted butter and cheese

8.   Instant foods like noodles, spaghetti, macaroni, and cornflakes

9.   Vegetables like cabbage, cauliflower, spinach, radish, beetroot, and coriander leaves

10.   Coconut water

11.   Drugs like sodium bicarbonate tablets, antacids, laxatives

12.   Non-vegetarian foods like meat, chicken, and animal innards like kidneys, liver and brain

13.   Seafoods like crab, lobster, oyster , shrimp, oily fish and dried fish

Practical Tips to Reduce Sodium in Food

1.   Restrict salt intake and avoid extra salt and baking soda in diet. Cook food without salt and add permitted amounts of salt separately. This is the best option to reduce salt intake and ensure consumption of the prescribed amount of salt in everyday diet.

2.   Avoid foods with high sodium content (as listed above).

3.   Do not serve salt and salty seasonings at the table or altogether remove the salt shaker from the dining table.

4.   Carefully read labels of commercially available packaged and processed foods. Look not only for salt but also for other sodium containing compounds. Carefully check the labels and choose "sodium-free" or "low-sodium" food products. Make sure however that potassium is not used to substitute sodium in these foods.

5.   Check sodium content of medications.

6.   Boil vegetables with high sodium content. Throw away the water. This can reduce sodium content in vegetables.

7.   To make a low salt diet tasty, one can add other spices and condiments such as garlic, onion, lemon juice, bay leaf, tamarind pulp, vinegar, cinnamon, cloves, nutmeg, black pepper, and cumin.

8.   **Caution!** Avoid the use of salt substitutes as they contain high amounts of potassium. High potassium content of salt substitutes can raise the potassium levels in blood to dangerous levels in CKD patients.

9.   Do not drink softened water. In the process of water softening, calcium is replaced by sodium. Water purified by reverse osmosis process is low in all minerals including sodium.

10.   While eating at restaurants, select foods that contain less sodium.

5. Potassium Restriction in Diet

Why are CKD patients advised to restrict potassium in diet?

Potassium is an important mineral in the body that is needed for the proper functioning of muscles and nerves and to keep the heart beat regular. Normally, the level of potassium in body is balanced by eating potassium containing foods and removal of excess potassium in the urine. Removal of excess potassium in the urine may be inadequate in a patient with chronic kidney disease and can lead to the accumulation of a high level of potassium in the blood (a condition known as hyperkalemia). The risk of hyperkalemia is less in patients undergoing peritoneal dialysis compared to those on hemodialysis. The risk differs in both groups because the process of dialysis is continuous in peritoneal dialysis while it is intermittent in hemodialysis.

High potassium levels can cause severe muscle weakness or an irregular heart rhythm that can be dangerous. When potassium is very high, the heart can stop beating unexpectedly and cause sudden death. High potassium levels can be life threatening without noticeable manifestations or symptoms (and therefore it is known as a silent killer).

To avoid serious consequences of high potassium, CKD patients are advised to restrict potassium in diet.

What is normal potassium level in blood? When is it considered high?

- The normal serum potassium (level of potassium in blood) is 3.5 mEq/L to 5.0 mEq/L.
- When the serum potassium is 5.0 to 6.0 mEq/L, dietary potassium needs to be limited.
- When the serum potassium is greater than 6.0 mEq/L, active medical intervention is needed to reduce it.
- A serum potassium greater than 7.0 mEq/L is life threatening and needs urgent treatment such as emergency dialysis.

Classification of food according to potassium content

To maintain proper control of potassium in blood, food intake must be modified as per the doctor's advice. On the basis of potassium contents, foods are classified into three different groups (high, medium, and low potassium containing foods).

High potassium   =   More than 200 mg/ 100 gms of food

Medium potassium   =   100 to 200 mg/ 100 gms of food

Low potassium   =   Less than 100 mg/ 100 gms of food

Foods with high potassium content

- **Fruits:** Fresh apricot, ripe banana, Chiku (Sapodilla), fresh coconut, custard apple, gooseberry, guava, kiwi fruit, ripe mango, oranges, papaya, peach, pomegranate and plum

- **Vegetables:** Broccoli, cluster beans, coriander, drumstick, mushroom, raw papaya, potato, pumpkin, spinach, sweet potato, tomatoes and yam

- **Dry fruits:** Almond, cashew nut, dates, dry figs, raisins and walnut

- **Cereals:** Wheat flour

- **Legumes:** Red and black beans and mung (monggo) beans

- **Non-vegetarian food:** Fish like anchovy and mackerel; shell fish like prawns, lobster and crabs; and beef

- **Drinks:** Coconut water, condensed milk, buffalo milk, cow milk, chocolate drinks, fresh fruit juices, soup, beer, wine and many aerated drinks

- **Miscellaneous:** Chocolate, chocolate cake, chocolate ice cream, Lona salt (salt substitute), potato chips and tomato sauce

Foods with Medium Potassium Content

- **Fruits:** Ripe cherries, grapes, lychees, pear, sweet lime and watermelon

- **Vegetables:** Beet root, raw banana, bitter gourd, cabbage, carrot, celery, cauliflower, French beans, okra (ladies finger), raw mango, onion, radish, green peas, sweet corn and safflower leaves

- **Cereals:** Barley, general purpose flour, noodles made from wheat flour, rice flakes (pressed rice) and wheat vermicelli

- **Non-vegetarian food:** Liver

- **Drinks:** Curd

Foods with Low Potassium Content

- **Fruits:** Apple, blackberries, lemon, pineapple and strawberries

- **Vegetables:** Bottle gourd, broad beans, capsicum, cucumber, garlic, lettuce and pointed gourd

- **Cereals:** Rice, rava and wheat semolina
- **Legumes:** Green peas
- **Non-vegetarian food:** Beef, lamb, pork, chicken and egg
- **Drinks:** Coca-cola, coffee, lemonade, lime juice in water, and soda
- **Miscellaneous:** Cloves, dried ginger, honey, mint leaves, mustard, nutmeg, black pepper and vinegar

Practical Tips to Reduce Potassium in Food

1. Take one fruit per day, preferably with low potassium.
2. Take one cup of tea or coffee per day.
3. Vegetables with potassium should be taken after reducing the amount of potassium (as mentioned below).
4. Avoid coconut water, fruit juices and foods with high potassium contents (as listed above).
5. Almost all food contains some potassium, so the key is to choose foods with a low potassium content when possible.
6. Restriction of potassium is necessary not only for predialysis CKD patients, but is also necessary even after initiating dialysis.

How does one reduce potassium content in vegetables?

- Peel and cut vegetables into small pieces.
- Wash vegetables with lukewarm water and put them in a large pot.
- Fill the pot with hot water (the quantity of water must be four to five times the volume of vegetables) and soak the vegetables for at least one hour.
- After soaking the vegetables for 2 - 3 hours, rinse them three times with warm water.
- Subsequently boil the vegetables with extra water. Discard the water.

- Cook the boiled vegetables as desired.

- Although you can reduce the amount of potassium in vegetables, it is still preferable to avoid high potassium containing vegetables or take them in small quantities.

- As vitamins are lost in cooked vegetables, vitamin supplements should be taken as per the doctor's advice.

Special tips for leaching potassium from potatoes

- Dicing, slicing or grating potatoes into smaller pieces is important. Maximizing the surface of the potatoes exposed to water by this method helps increase potassium loss from the potatoes.

- The temperature of the water used to either soak or boil the potatoes makes the difference.

- Using large amounts of water to soak or boil potatoes is helpful.

6. Phosphorus Restriction in Diet

Why must CKD patients take a low phosphorus diet?

- Phosphorus is a mineral essential to keep bones strong and healthy. Excess phosphorus present in food is removed from the body by urine excretion. This maintains blood phosphorus levels.

- The normal value of phosphorus in blood is 4.0 to 5.5 mg/dl.

- Patients with CKD cannot eliminate the extra phosphorus taken in food so the blood level rises. This increased phosphorus drains out calcium from the bones making them weak.

- Increase in phosphorus level can lead to many problems like itching, weakness of muscles and bones, bone pains, bone stiffness and joint pains. The stiffness of bone results in increased susceptibility to fracture.

What foods containing high phosphorus should be reduced or avoided?

Foods containing high phosphorous include:

- Milk and dairy products: cheese, chocolate, condensed milk, ice cream, milk shake.

- Dry fruits: cashew nuts, almonds, pistachios, dry coconut, walnuts.

- Cold drinks: dark colas, beer.

- Carrot, corn, groundnut, fresh peas, sweet potato.

- Animal protein: meats, chicken, fish and egg.

7. High Vitamin and Fiber Intake

CKD patients generally suffer from an inadequate supply of vitamins during the predialysis period due to poor appetite, and an overly restricted diet in the attempt to delay progression of renal disease. Certain vitamins – especially water soluble vitamins B, vitamin C and folic acid – are lost during dialysis.

To compensate for inadequate intake or loss of these vitamins, CKD patients usually need supplementation of water-soluble vitamins and trace elements. High fiber intake is beneficial in CKD. Patients are therefore advised to take more fresh vegetables and fruits rich in vitamin and fibers while avoiding those with high potassium content.

Designing the Daily Food

For CKD patients daily food intake and water intake are planned and charted out by the dietitian in accordance with the advice of the nephrologist.

Common principles for the diet plan are:

1. **Water and liquid food intake:** Fluid intake should be restricted according to the doctor's advice. Daily weight chart must be maintained. Any inappropriate gain in weight may indicate increased fluid intake.

2. **Carbohydrate:** To ensure that the body gets adequate calories, the CKD patient can take sugar or glucose containing food along with cereals provided he/she is not diabetic.

3. **Protein:** Lean meat, milk, cereals, legumes, eggs and chicken are the main sources of protein. CKD patients who are not on dialysis are advised to limit dietary protein to < 0.8 grams/kg body weight/day. Once dialysis is started, dietary intake can be increased to 1-1.2 grams/kg body weight/day.

   Patients undergoing peritoneal dialysis may need dietary proteins as high as 1.5 grams/kg body weight per day. While animal proteins contain all essential amino acids (hence are called complete proteins or proteins with high biologic value) and would be ideal, they should be limited especially in patients not yet on dialysis because they may accelerate the progression of CKD.

4. **Fat:** Fats may be taken in as an energy source since they are a good source of calories. Monounsaturated and polyunsaturated fats in the form of olive oil, safflower oil, canola oil or soybean oil may be taken in limited quantities. Avoid saturated fats such as those found in animal lards.

5. **Salt:** Most patients are advised to take a low salt diet. It is good to observe a "no added salt" diet. Look at food labels and go for low sodium foods but make sure that salt substitutes containing high amounts of potassium are also avoided. Check food labels for other foods containing sodium such as sodium bicarbonate (baking powder) and avoid them.

6. **Cereals:** Rice or rice products like flattened rice can be taken. To avoid monotony of taste one can rotate intake of various cereals like wheat, rice, sago, semolina, all purpose flour, and cornflakes. Small quantities of corn and barley can be taken.

7. **Vegetables:** Vegetables with low potassium can be liberally taken. But vegetables with high potassium must be processed to remove potassium before consumption. To improve taste, lemon juice can be added.

8. **Fruits:** Fruits with low potassium content like apple, papaya and berry can be taken but only once a day. On the day of dialysis, patients can take any one fruit. Fruit juice and coconut water must be avoided.

9. **Milk and milk products:** Milk and milk products such as milk, yogurt and cheese contain large amounts of phosphorus and need to be limited. Other dairy foods that have lower amounts of phosphorus include butter, cream cheese, ricotta cheese, sherbets and nondairy whipped toppings may be taken instead.

10. **Cold drinks:** Avoid dark colored sodas as they have a high phosphorus content. Do not take fruit juice or coconut water because of the potentially high potassium content.

11. **Dry fruits:** Dry fruits, groundnut, sesame seeds, fresh or dry coconut must be avoided.

Glossary

Glossary

Acute kidney failure (injury): A condition in which there is sudden or rapid loss of kidney functions. This type of kidney damage is temporary and usually reversible.

Anemia: It is a medical condition in which hemoglobin is reduced in blood. Anemia leads to weakness, fatigue and shortness of breath on exertion. Anemia is common in CKD and occurs due to decreased erythropoietin production by kidney.

Automated peritoneal dialysis (APD): See CCPD.

Arteriovenous fistula (AV Fistula): It means creating a connection between artery and vein surgically, usually in the forearm. In an AV fistula a large amount of blood with high pressure enters into the vein causing dilatation of the vein. The enlarged dilated veins allow easy repeated needle insertion required for hemodialysis. AV fistula is the most common and the best method of vascular access for long term hemodialysis.

Artificial kidney: See dialyzer.

Benign prostatic hypertrophy (BPH): It is common for the prostate gland to become enlarged as a man ages. BPH is a non-cancerous prostatic enlargement in elderly males which compresses the urethra, blocks urine stream and causes problems in urination.

Blood pressure: It is the force exerted by circulating blood on the walls of blood vessels as the heart pumps out blood. Blood pressure is one of the principal vital signs and its measurement consists of two numbers. The first number indicates systolic blood pressure which measures the maximum pressure exerted when heart contracts. The second number indicates diastolic pressure, a measurement taken between beats, when the heart is at rest.

Brain death: Brain death: It is a severe and permanent damage to brain that does not respond with any medical or surgical treatment. In brain death, the body's respiration and blood circulation are artificially maintained.

Cadaveric kidney transplantation: See deceased kidney transplantation.

Calcium: The most abundant mineral in the body, essential for the development and maintenance of strong bones and teeth. Milk and milk products like yogurt and cheese are rich natural sources of calcium.

Catheter for hemodialysis: It is a long, flexible hollow tube with two lumens. Blood is withdrawn from one lumen, enters the dialysis circuit for purification, and is returned to the body via the other lumen. Insertion of double lumen catheter is the most common and effective method for emergency and temporary hemodialysis.

Continuous ambulatory peritoneal dialysis (CAPD): CAPD is a form of dialysis that can be carried out by a person at home without the use of a machine. In this type of dialysis, fluid is exchanged at regular intervals throughout the day, i.e. 24-hours a day, seven days a week.

Continuous cycling peritoneal dialysis (CCPD): CCPD or Automated peritoneal dialysis (APD) is a form of continuous peritoneal dialysis carried out at home every day with an automated cycler machine. In CCPD, a machine performs fluid exchanges while the patient is sleeping at night. In this process the machine automatically fills and drains the dialysis solution from the abdomen.

Creatinine and urea: These are breakdown or waste products of protein metabolism. These substances are removed by kidneys. The usual level of serum creatinine is 0.8 to 1.4 mg% and that of urea is 2 to 4 mg%. In kidney failure the level of urea and creatinine in blood rises.

Chronic kidney disease (CKD): Gradual progressive and irreversible loss of kidney function over several months to years is called chronic kidney disease. In this non- curable disease, kidney function reduces slowly and continuously. After a long period it reduces to a stage where the kidney stops working almost completely. This advanced and life threatening stage of the disease is called End Stage Kidney Disease ESKD.

Cystoscopy: A diagnostic procedure in which the doctor looks inside the bladder and the urethra using a thin, lighted instrument called a cystoscope.

Deceased (cadaveric) kidney transplantation: It is a surgical procedure in which a healthy kidney donated by a person with brain death is transplanted in a patient with chronic kidney disease.

Diabetic kidney disease (nephropathy): Long-standing diabetes causes damage to small blood vessels of the kidney. This damage initially causes loss of protein in urine. Subsequently it causes hypertension, swelling and then gradual and progressive damage to the kidney. Finally, progressive deterioration leads to severe kidney failure (End stage kidney disease). This diabetes induced kidney problem is known as diabetic kidney disease. Diabetic kidney disease is the most common cause of chronic kidney disease, accounting for 40-45 percent of new cases of CKD.

Dialysis: It is an artificial process by which waste products and unwanted water is removed from the body in patients with kidney failure.

Dialyzer: An artificial kidney that filters blood and removes wastes and extra water from the body in the process of hemodialysis.

Diuretics: Drugs that increase the production of urine and increases excretion of water in the form of urine which helps to lose water from body. Diuretics are also called "water pills."

Dry weight: It is the weight of a person after all excess fluid is removed by dialysis.

Dwell time: During peritoneal dialysis, the period for which PD fluid remains in the abdomen is called the dwell time. During dwell time the process of purification takes place.

eGFR: The eGFR (estimated Glomerular Filtration Rate) is a number which is calculated from blood creatinine level and other information. eGFR measures how well kidneys are working and its normal value is 90 or more. The eGFR test is useful for the diagnosis, grading of stages and monitoring the progression of CKD.

Electrolytes: There are many minerals like sodium, potassium, calcium in the blood stream that regulate important function of the body. These chemicals are called electrolytes. As the kidney keeps the electrolyte concentrations constant in blood, in patients with kidney diseases, blood is tested to check electrolyte levels.

Endstage kidney disease (ESKD): Advanced stage of chronic kidney disease (Stage 5 CKD) is known as endstage kidney disease (ESKD) or end stage renal disease (ESRD). At this stage of CKD there is complete or almost complete failure of the kidneys. ESKD patients need treatment, such as dialysis or transplantation, to lead a fairly normal life.

Erythropoietin (EPO): It is a hormone produced by the kidneys that promotes the formation of red blood cells by the bone marrow. If the kidneys are damaged, they are not able to produce enough erythropoietin resulting in decrease in the formation of red blood cells which leads to anemia. Erythropoietin is available as an injectable medication for the treatment of anemia due to kidney failure.

Exchange: It means one complete cycle of peritoneal dialysis, consisting of three stages. The first stage is inflow of dialysis fluid in the abdomen. In the second stage, the fluid remains in the abdomen for several hours allowing excess fluid and toxins to move from the blood to the dialysis fluid (also called dwell). The third stage is outflow of the dialysis fluid.

Extracorporeal shock wave lithotripsy (ESWL): It is a modality in which highly concentrated shock waves produced by a lithotriptor machine break up urinary stones. The stones break down into small particles and are easily passed through the urinary tract in urine. ESWL is an effective and widely used treatment modality for kidney stones.

Fistula: See arteriovenous fistula.

Graft: A type of access for long term hemodialysis. Graft is a short piece of synthetic soft tube which joins a vein and an artery in the arm. Needles are inserted in this graft during hemodialysis treatment.

Hemodialysis: Most popular modality to treat kidney failure. In hemodialysis blood is purified with the help of dialysis machine and an artificial kidney (dialyzer).

Hemoglobin: It is a protein molecule in red blood cells that carries oxygen from the lungs to the body tissues and returns carbon dioxide from the tissues to the lungs. Hemoglobin is measured by blood test and its reduced value is referred as anemia.

Hyperkalemia: Normal serum potassium levels are between 3.5 and 5.0 mEq/L. Hyperkalemia is a condition characterized by elevated levels of potassium in the blood. Hyperkalemia is common in kidney failure, can be life threatening, and requires urgent medical treatment.

Hypertension: It is the term used to describe high blood pressure.

Immunosuppressant Drug: Medications that suppress or decrease the body's immune system and prevent the body from rejecting a transplanted organ.

Intravenous urogram (IVU): It is an investigation where a series of x-rays of the urinary system is taken after injecting an intravenous iodine containing dye. This test gives information about function of the kidney and structure of the urinary tract.

Kidney biopsy: A procedure to get a small piece of kidney tissue with a needle so that it can be examined under a microscope for the diagnosis of the disease.

Kidney failure: Condition in which deterioration in kidney function leads to inadequate filtration of toxins and waste products from the blood. It is characterized by an increase in urea and creatinine levels in blood.

Microalbuminuria: Refers to the appearance of small but abnormal amounts of albumin in urine. Its presence indicates early onset of diabetic kidney disease.

Micturating cystourethrogram: See voiding cystouretehrogram.

Nephron: The functional unit of the kidney responsible for the actual purification and filtration of the blood. Each kidney contains about one million nephrons.

Nephrologist: A physician specialized in kidney diseases.

Nephrotic syndrome: Kidney problem that is seen more frequently in children characterized by loss of protein in urine (more than 3.5 grams per day), low blood protein levels, high cholesterol levels, and swelling.

Paired kidney transplantation: Many patients with endstage kidney disease have healthy and willing potential kidney donors with an incompatible blood type or tissue cross match.Paired kidney donation is the strategy that allows the exchange of living donor kidneys between two incompatible donor/recipient pairs to create two compatible pairs.

Peritoneal dialysis: It is an effective treatment modality for kidney failure. In this process of purification, dialysis fluid is introduced into the abdominal cavity through a special catheter. This fluid removes waste products and extra water from the blood. Fluid is removed from the abdomen after a variable period of time, and discarded.

Peritonitis: It is an infection inside the abdominal cavity. Peritonitis is a common complication of peritoneal dialysis and can be life threatening, if not treated.

Phosphorus: Phosphorus is the second most-abundant mineral found in the body, next only to calcium. It works with calcium to build strong bones and teeth. Meats, nuts, milk, eggs, cereals are phosphorus rich foods.

Polycystic kidney disease (PKD): PKD is the most common genetic disorder of the kidney, characterized by the growth of numerous cysts (fluid sacs) in the kidneys. It is among the leading causes of chronic kidney disease.

Potassium: It is a very important mineral in the body needed for the proper function of nerves, heart and muscles. Fresh fruit, fruit juices, coconut water and dry fruits are rich sources of potassium.

Pre-emptive kidney transplantation: Kidney transplantation is usually carried out after a variable period of dialysis therapy. A kidney transplant done before the initiation of maintenance dialysis is a pre-emptive kidney transplant.

Proteins: They are one of the three main classes of food that build, repair and maintain body tissues. Pulses, milk, eggs and animal foods are rich sources of protein.

Proteinuria: Presence of abnormally high levels of protein in urine.

Rejection: The process in which the body recognizes that a transplanted organ is not its own and tries to destroy it.

Semipermeable membrane: A membrane that selectively allows certain dissolved substances and fluid to pass through, while holding back the others. Membrane is a thin natural tissue or artificial material.

Sodium: A mineral in the body that regulates blood pressure and blood volume. The most common form of sodium in food is sodium chloride, which is table salt.

Trans-urethral Resection of the Prostate (TURP): It is the standard treatment for benign prostatic hyperplasia (BPH) performed by urologists. In this minimally-invasive surgical treatment, an instrument called a cystoscope is passed through the urethra and the prostate gland blocking the urine flow is removed.

Ultrasound: It is a painless diagnostic test that uses high frequency sound waves to create an image of the organs or structures inside the body. Ultrasound is a simple, useful and safe test that provides valuable information such as the size of kidney, obstruction to urine flow, and the presence of cyst, stone and tumors.

Urologist: A surgeon specialized in kidney diseases.

Vesicoureteral reflux (VUR): It is a condition with an abnormal backward flow (reflux) of urine from the bladder toward the ureters and possibly up to the kidneys. This is an anatomic and functional disorder that can happen either on one or both sides. VUR is the major cause of urinary tract infection, high blood pressure and kidney failure in children.

Voiding cystourethrogram: A procedure used to outline the anatomy of the lower urinary tract (bladder and urethra) by catheterizing a patient and introducing solution (dye) which can be seen on X-ray films. The patient is asked to void urine and X-rays are taken

Abbreviations

ACE	:	Angiotensin Converting Enzyme
ADPKD	:	Autosomal Dominant Polycystic Kidney Disease
AGN	:	Acute Glomerulonephritis
AKI	:	Acute Kidney Injury
APD	:	Automated Peritoneal Dialysis
ARB	:	Angiotensin Receptor Blockers
ARF	:	Acute Renal Failure
AV Fistula	:	Arterio Venous Fistula
BP	:	Blood Pressure
BPH	:	Benign Prostatic Hypertrophy/Hyperplasia
BUN	:	Blood Urea Nitrogen
CAPD	:	Continuous Ambulatory Peritoneal Dialysis
CCPD	:	Continuous Cycling Peritoneal Dialysis
CKD	:	Chronic Kidney Disease
CRF	:	Chronic Renal Failure
DKD	:	Diabetic Kidney Disease
DM	:	Diabetes Mellitus
DMSA	:	Dimercaptosuccinic Acid
eGFR	:	Estimated Glomerular Filtration Rate
EPO	:	Erythropoietin
ESKD	:	End Stage Kidney Disease
ESRD	:	End Stage Renal Disease
ESWL	:	Extracorporeal Shock Wave Lithotripsy
GFR	:	Glomerular Filtration Rate
HD	:	Hemodialysis

IDDM	:	Insulin Dependent Diabetes Mellitus
IJV	:	Internal Jugular Vein
IPD	:	Intermittent Peritoneal Dialysis
IVU/IVP	:	Intravenous Urography/Pyelography
MA	:	Microalbuminuria
MCU	:	Micturating Cysto Urethrogram
MRI	:	Magnetic Resonance Imaging
NIDDM	:	Non-Insulin Dependent Diabetes
NSAID	:	Non-Steroidal Anti-Inflammatory Drug
PCNL	:	Percutanous Nephrolitomy
PD	:	Peritoneal Dialysis
PKD	:	Polycystic Kidney Disease
PSA	:	Prostate Specific Antigen
PUV	:	Posterior Urethral Valves
RBC	:	Red Blood Cells
RRT	:	Renal Replacement Therapy
TB	:	Tuberculosis
TIBC	:	Total Iron Binding Capacity
TURP	:	Trans Urethral Resection of Prostrate
UTI	:	Urinary Tract Infection
VCUG	:	Voiding Cysto Urethrogram
VUR	:	Vesicoureteral Reflux
WBC	:	White Blood Cells

Common Blood Tests for Kidney Patients

Commonly used laboratory blood tests for kidney patients and their reference ranges are summarized below.

Test	Conventional units	Conversion factor	SI units
Blood Tests for Kidney Function			
Blood urea nitrogen	8 - 20 mg/dl	0.36	2.9 - 7.1 mmol/L
Creatinine Male	0.7 - 1.3 mg/dl	88.4	68 - 118 mcmd/L
Female	0.6 - 1.2 mg/dl	88.4	50 - 100 mcmd/L
eGFR	90 - 120 ml/min	--	--
Blood Tests for Anemia			
Hemoglobin Male	13.5 - 17.0 g/dl	10	136 - 175 g/L
Female	12.0 - 15.5 g/dl	10	120 - 155 g/L
Hematocrit Male	41 - 53%	0.01	0.41 - 0.53
Female	36 - 48%	0.01	0.36 - 0.48
Iron total	50 - 175 mcg/dl	0.18	9 - 31 mcmol/L
Iron-binding capacity total	240 - 450 mcg/dl	0.18	45 - 82 mcmol/L
Transferrin	190 - 375 mg/dl	0.01	1.9 - 3.75 g/L
Transferrin saturation	20 - 50 %	--	--
Ferritin Male	16 - 300 ng/ml	2.25	36 - 675 pmol/L
Female	10 - 200 ng/ml	2.25	22.5 - 450 pmol/L

Test	Conventional units	Conversion factor	SI units
Blood Tests for Electrolytes and Metabolic Bone Diseases			
Sodium (Na)	135 - 145 mEq/L	1.0	135 - 145 mmol/L
Potassium (K)	3.5 - 5.0 mEq/L	1.0	3.5 - 5.0 mmol/L
Chloride (Cl)	101 - 112 mEq/L	1	101- 112 mmol/L
Calcium ionized	4.4 - 5.2 mg/dL	0.25	1.10 - 1.30 mmol/L
Calcium total	8.5 - 10.5 mg/dl	0.25	2.2 - 2.8 mmol/L
Phosphorus inorganic	2.5 - 4.5 mg/dl	0.32	0.8 - 1.45 mmol/L
Magnesium	1.8 - 3 mg/dl	0.41	0.75 - 1.25 mmol/L
Bicarbonate	22 - 28 mEq/L	1	22 - 28 mmol/L
Uric acid Male	2.4 - 7.4 mg/dl	59.48	140 - 440 mcmol/L
Female	1.4 - 5.8 mg/dl	59.48	80 - 350 mcmol/L
PTH	11 - 54 pg/ml	0.11	1.2 - 5.7 pmol/L
Blood Tests for General Health			
Protein Total	6.0 - 8.0 g/dl	10	60 - 80 g/L
Albumin	3.4 - 4.7 g/dl	10	34 - 47 g/L
Cholesterol total	100 - 220 mg/dl	0.03	3.0 - 6.5 mmol/L
Blood sugar fasting	60 - 110 mg/dl	0.055	3.3 - 6.1 mmol/L
Blood Tests for Liver Function			
Bilirubin Total	0.1 - 1.2 mg/dl	17.1	2 - 21 mcmol/L
Direct	0.1 - 0.5 mg/dl	17.1	<8 mcmol/L
Indirect	0.1 - 0.7 mg/dl	17.1	<12 mcmol/L
Alanine transaminase (SGPT)	7 - 56 unit/L	0.02	0.14 - 1.12 mckat/L
Aspartate transaminase (SGOT)	0 - 35 units/L	0.02	0 - 0.58 mckat/L
Alkaline phosphatase	41- 133 units/L	0.02	0.7 - 2.2 mckat/L

Index

Printed in Great Britain
by Amazon

47639212R00136